T'ai Chi For Dummies

Cheat Sheet

Following the Principles of T'ai Chi

- **Slow down.** This is the Grand Ultimate Principle because you begin to find all the benefits of T'ai Chi if you go slowly.
- **Take it easy.** Forcing things is an antithesis in T'ai Chi. Physical and mental stress make you tense up and get all the forms wrong.
- **Think in curves.** Movement in T'ai Chi is always curved and circular, never straight and linear. This allows one movement to flow seamlessly to the next and promotes a better flow of your *chi* (energy).
- **Be simple.** Live fully. Live naturally. And be simple at your core.
- **Sink lower.** In other words, let your knees relax and bend at the joint. This grounds you, lets energy flow from the earth into your body, and allows you to overpower your opponent by getting beneath his or her energy and center.
- **Balance your movements.** Just as all things in the universe are reciprocal, T'ai Chi is about balancing your moves — for example, forward and back, weight-bearing and non-weight-bearing, and reach and pull back. This is based on the ancient Chinese philosophy of *yin and yang,* in which all living things are opposing yet complementary.
- **Stay balanced.** Both physically and mentally, good balance is essential to good T'ai Chi — and to life.
- **Move the whole package.** Your whole body, not just a wrist or leg, is a part of T'ai Chi movement. Think action-reaction. Think flow.
- **Go with the flow.** Think smooth as silk. Move and think as if you are on wheels, not herky-jerky with breaks. That cuts into your energy flow.
- **Stay rooted.** Always feel that you are firmly planted on the ground. This applies not only to T'ai Chi but also to life — what else is new?

Words to Note

- **Chi:** Otherwise known as "life energy," this is the life force that pulses through your body and keeps you vital. Blocked chi can cause sickness or unhappiness.
- **Meridians:** Also known as "energy pathways," these are the streets, roads, and byways in your body through which energy flows. These pathways can get kinked from poor health and stress and can therefore block energy from flowing through your body.
- **Dan Tien:** Literally meaning "elixir field," this area is located approximately between your navel and pubic bone and is a storehouse of body energy.
- **Yin and yang:** The terms for opposites that are opposing yet complementary. A concept used throughout all of T'ai Chi and Qigong.

T'ai Chi For Dummies®

Basic T'ai Chi and Qigong Movements

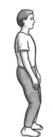

T'ai Chi Posture

Bow Stance

Hold Balloon

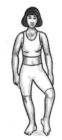

Centering Step

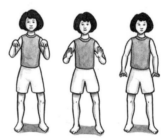

Commencement

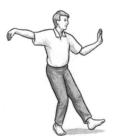

Single Whip

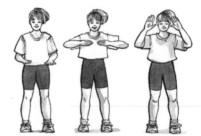

Standing Like a Tree (Embrace the Tree hands)

A Wise Quote to Live By

Flow with whatever may happen and let your mind be free: Stay centered by accepting what you are doing. This is the ultimate.

— *Chuang-Tzu,* The Writings of Chuang-Tzu

Wiley, the Wiley Publishing logo, For Dummies, the Dummies Man logo, the For Dummies Bestselling Book Series logo and all related trade dress are trademarks or registered trademarks of Wiley Publishing, Inc. All other trademarks are property of their respective owners.

For Dummies: Bestselling Book Series for Beginners

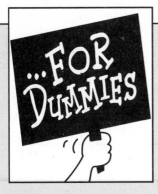

TM

BESTSELLING BOOK SERIES

References for the Rest of Us!®

Do you find that traditional reference books are overloaded with technical details and advice you'll never use? Do you postpone important life decisions because you just don't want to deal with them? Then our *For Dummies*® business and general reference book series is for you.

For Dummies business and general reference books are written for those frustrated and hard-working souls who know they aren't dumb, but find that the myriad of personal and business issues and the accompanying horror stories make them feel helpless. *For Dummies* books use a lighthearted approach, a down-to-earth style, and even cartoons and humorous icons to dispel fears and build confidence. Lighthearted but not lightweight, these books are perfect survival guides to solve your everyday personal and business problems.

> *"More than a publishing phenomenon, 'Dummies' is a sign of the times."*
>
> — The New York Times

> *"...you won't go wrong buying them."*
>
> — Walter Mossberg, Wall Street Journal, on For Dummies books

> *"A world of detailed and authoritative information is packed into them..."*
>
> — U.S. News and World Report

Already, millions of satisfied readers agree. They have made For Dummies the #1 introductory level computer book series and a best-selling business book series. They have written asking for more. So, if you're looking for the best and easiest way to learn about business and other general reference topics, look to For Dummies to give you a helping hand.

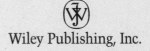

Wiley Publishing, Inc.

T'ai Chi

FOR

DUMMIES®

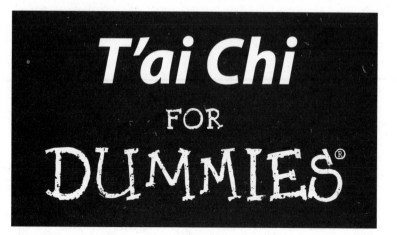

by Therese Iknoian
with Manny Fuentes

WILEY

Wiley Publishing, Inc.

T'ai Chi For Dummies®

Published by
Wiley Publishing, Inc.
909 Third Avenue
New York, NY 10022
www.wiley.com

Copyright © 2001 by Wiley Publishing, Inc., Indianapolis, Indiana

Published by Wiley Publishing, Inc., Indianapolis, Indiana

Published simultaneously in Canada

For general information on our other products and services or to obtain technical support, please contact our Customer Care Department within the U.S. at 800-762-2974, outside the U.S. at 317-572-3993, or fax 317-572-4002.

Wiley also publishes its books in a variety of electronic formats. Some content that appears in print may not be available in electronic books.

Library of Congress Cataloging-in-Publication Data:

Library of Congress Control Number: 2001089345

ISBN: 0-7645-5351-8

Manufactured in the United States of America

10 9 8 7 6 5 4

3B/RV/QT/QT/IN

About the Authors

Along with degrees in journalism and exercise physiology, **Therese Iknoian** has a long reputation as a fitness author and instructor. She spent a decade as a newspaper reporter before launching a freelance career specializing in sports/fitness writing and instruction and earning her master's degree in exercise physiology. She has been a nationally ranked race walker and is an internationally published freelance health and fitness writer whose work has appeared in dozens of national publications. She is also a partner in GearTrends LLC — www.GearTrends.com — the premier sports/outdoor product information Web site, and in SNEWS, an outdoor/fitness trade newsletter. Her other Web site, award-winning Total Fitness Network — www.TotalFitnessNetwork.com — is filled with her stories about all areas of fitness and training.

Long known by some as "The Walking Woman," Therese Iknoian's first books — *Fitness Walking* (Human Kinetics, 1995) and *Walking Fast* (Human Kinetics, 1998) — were on that topic, as were two instruction/music audiotapes. She has also developed fitness, running, and walking programs for several international companies. She broke new ground in 2000, authoring *Mind-Body Fitness For Dummies,* published by Wiley Publishing, Inc.

Therese, a sought-after lecturer and trainer, is an American College of Sports Medicine-certified Health/Fitness Instructor, a gold-certified ACE instructor, and a USA Track & Field Level II-certified coach who focuses on working with kids. As a race walker, she was ranked 24th among all women in the country in 1995, and she broke several age-group records. Therese ran her first marathon in 2000 and qualified for the Boston 2001 Marathon, where she also collected a finisher's medal. In 1999, her team placed 3rd in the corporate division in the New York Hi-Tec Adventure Race.

These days, if Therese isn't writing, she's running, mountain biking, or looking for the next fitness adventure challenge. Or she's sitting beside the creek behind her house in the Sierra foothills enjoying the sounds of quiet.

Manny Fuentes is a clinical exercise physiologist in the cardiopulmonary rehabilitation department of Lafayette General Medical Center in Lafayette, Louisiana. He holds a bachelor's degree in exercise science and a master's degree in health services. He is certified as an Exercise Specialist by the American College of Sports Medicine and also holds the ACSM Advanced Personal Trainer certificate of enhanced qualifications. Additionally, he holds the National Strength and Conditioning Association's Certified Strength and Conditioning Specialist credential.

Manny began his martial arts training in 1984, studying Tae Kwon Do in college. A back injury limited his ability to progress in Tae Kwon Do, and in 1988 he began the study of Hsing-I, followed by training in Yang-style T'ai Chi. He has taught T'ai Chi to a wide range of populations including senior citizens, college students, and cardiac and pulmonary patients as well as individuals in treatment for chronic pain. He has taught in a variety of settings such as hospitals, church halls, college campuses, and parks. Manny not only lectures to health and exercise professionals on using T'ai Chi, but he also combines his other areas of expertise to provide instruction on additional health-related topics such as meditation, stress management, and exercise program design.

Dedication

From Therese: To my parents, who instilled in me the belief that everything was possible, and to my husband, with whom I fulfilled a dream of living in the mountains surrounded by utmost beauty, energy, and stillness.

From Manny: To my father and my late mother, my first teachers whose lessons still resonate today.

Authors' Acknowledgments

From Therese: Thanks, perhaps oddly enough, must go partly to this book itself for coaxing me to more deeply explore T'ai Chi and its Taoist principles that I find so insightful and perceptive. This and my previous book, *Mind-Body Fitness For Dummies,* have allowed me to explore mindful areas of fitness on a much deeper level and to share those discoveries with others, as well as grow and incorporate them into my lifestyle.

I must also acknowledge and gratefully thank my collaborator Manny for always being johnny-on-the-spot with writing, comments, responses, wise words, and even a little humor whenever needed. No other collaborator could have gone so far beyond the call of duty as he did and been so knowledgeable and giving with his expertise. We both learned from each other, bending one way or the other as needed as we hammered out issues and presentation styles.

I also can't ever thank enough my husband, Michael, for putting up with my occasional late nights or any obsessing I sometimes did about getting something right or meeting a deadline. Yes, a well-timed reminder, even to me, to breathe comes in handy.

And, as always, my parents Richard and Roxy continue to earn mountains of thanks for helping to get me to this place of contentment and for providing me their support, their constant encouragement, and their love.

From Manny: When I sat down to write my acknowledgment of and thanks to all the people who helped me get to the point of this book, I was reminded of just how interconnected we all are and how much we all need and mean to one another. First, I want to thank Therese for the invitation to co-author this book. She is a consummate professional, and I commend her ability to work with someone as right-brain-oriented as myself. She was the driving force behind this book and deserves the lion's share of the credit. I thank her for her guidance and patience.

Thanks also to Tom Sattler for getting me on the agenda for the American College of Sports Medicine Health & Fitness Summit where Therese and I met. He is a good friend and fantastic speaker, and I remain his biggest fan. My thanks to my Tae Kwon Do instructor, Mike Smith, for teaching me that there is more to martial arts than punching and kicking. I will be forever indebted to Noah West, my instructor in T'ai Chi and Hsing-I, whose talents far surpass my own. I am grateful, also, to all my students for the learning and growth they have given me, and to my bosses at Iberia Medical Center and Lafayette General Medical Center for the opportunity to teach T'ai Chi. I am grateful to my coworkers Judy, Sharon, and Stephanie who have been so supportive during the writing of this book. And finally, my thanks to Rebecca for her support, patience, and tolerance throughout the writing.

Publisher's Acknowledgments

We're proud of this book; please send us your comments through our online registration form located at www.dummies.com/register.

Some of the people who helped bring this book to market include the following:

Acquisitions, Editorial, and Media Development

Project Editor: Tonya Maddox

Acquisitions Editors: Stacy Collins, Tracy Boggier

Copy Editor: Mary Fales

Technical Editor: Yaj Rabnud

Editorial Manager: Jennifer Ehrlich

Editorial Assistant: Jennifer Young

Cover Photos: ©Arthur Tilley/FPG

Production

Project Coordinators: Jennifer Bingham, Maridee Ennis

Layout and Graphics: Amy Adrian, Joyce Haughey, Barry Offringa, Jacque Schneider, Betty Schulte, Julie Trippetti

Special Art: Lisa S. Reed and Kelly R. Pulley, Visual Diner Studio

Proofreaders: John Greenough, TECHBOOKS Production Services

Indexer: TECHBOOKS Production Services

Special Help
Billie A. Williams, Christine Meloy Beck, Linda Brandon, Kristin A. Cocks, Kathleen A. Dobie

---

Publishing and Editorial for Consumer Dummies
Diane Graves Steele, Vice President and Publisher, Consumer Dummies
Joyce Pepple, Acquisitions Director, Consumer Dummies
Kristin A. Cocks, Product Development Director, Consumer Dummies
Michael Spring, Vice President and Publisher, Travel
Brice Gosnell, Publishing Director, Travel
Suzanne Jannetta, Editorial Director, Travel

Publishing for Technology Dummies
Richard Swadley, Vice President and Executive Group Publisher
Andy Cummings, Vice President and Publisher

Composition Services
Gerry Fahey, Vice President of Production Services
Debbie Stailey, Director of Composition Services

Contents at a Glance

Cartoons at a Glance

By Rich Tennant

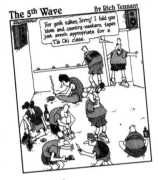

page 43

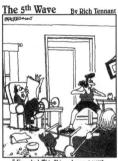

"I'm glad T'ai Chi relaxes you!"

page 73

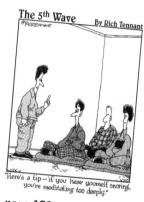

"Here's a tip—if you hear yourself snoring, you're meditating too deeply."

page 183

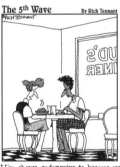

"Sandy says she's going to repulse the monkey. I can only hope it has something to do with her T'ai Chi routine or we could be in trouble with the local zoo."

page 215

"I'm always endeavoring to become one with all things, however I'm going to make an exception with this fish casserole."

page 9

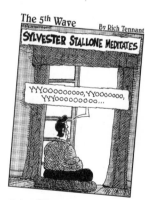

page 265

Cartoon Information:
Fax: 978-546-7747
E-Mail: richtennant@the5thwave.com
World Wide Web: www.the5thwave.com

Table of Contents

Introduction

. . . .

*W*hat Westerners do for recreation, sports, or exercise has changed greatly in the last few decades. Even three decades ago, sitting cross-legged on the floor to meditate or doing slow and mindful Asian-oriented movement was something that only the anti-establishment hippy types did. (Do you recall that kind of name-calling?) Today, the establishment is joining them in these less-traditional activities.

What's interesting is the use of the terms "less traditional" to describe T'ai Chi and Qigong. The Chinese and other Eastern cultures consider things like meditating or moving slowly in a park to be pretty darn traditional, but they've considered jumping around a room to disco music, taking your pulse, and running or walking around city streets for fitness to be pretty odd.

But times are changing. Westerners have become more tolerant, accepting, and open of Eastern practices, and Easterners have become the same of Western practices. Each type of activity has its rewards.

Practicing T'ai Chi and other internal martial arts can give a boost to your health and your workout for several reasons:

✔ You find out how to slow down instead of always going faster and harder.

✔ You can capture the essence of another culture and its traditions and, in turn, personally expand your horizons.

✔ Your body gets stronger and more balanced in fine ways that many other forms of movement miss.

✔ Your mind begins to understand how to be with itself and its own thoughts.

About This Book

Transferring the essence of T'ai Chi and Qigong to the printed page is a tough row to hoe. T'ai Chi and Qigong movement is all about flow and connection with an emphasis on three dimensions, yet the printed page is flat and one-dimensional.

Transmitting the true heart of these movements from written descriptions and some drawings is a great challenge. In this book, I am honored to take on that challenge, which forced a lot of contemplation about how best to present the information. This book also presents a nontraditional and light-hearted style, which is contradictory to what is known as traditional T'ai Chi! This movement art is about seriousness and contemplation.

Thus, I use this guide as a place to present simple T'ai Chi definitions and basic movements and forms. And the light-hearted and sometimes humorous Dummies style is the perfect way to break down the barriers and intimidation that Westerners may feel when reading deeply philosophical T'ai Chi tomes. In fact, I choose some rather nontraditional ways to present some sections, ones that took some work to convince my collaborator Manny Fuentes to go along with! You see, I am someone who is an all-around movement artist and athlete who isn't as deeply imbedded in the Asian cultures and the traditions of T'ai Chi as someone who is only an instructor or student of the martial arts. Therefore, I am perhaps able to think outside the box, looking for ways that are perhaps less intimidating. I hope that I succeed.

Why You Need This Book

This book serves to open up the sacred gates behind which T'ai Chi and Qigong sometimes remain locked.

Whether you are already dabbling in T'ai Chi or you are thinking about trying it, this book lays out definitions and breaks down movements in ways that some instructors who aren't well-versed in Western learning styles are necessarily best at. I had an instructor who sort of looked at me funny every time I asked a question about what we were doing. One doesn't traditionally question a movement or the teacher. But it was important to me to know the why or the concept behind a movement so I was able to fully integrate it into my body and feel its essence.

That's what this book does for you. When you ask questions, it gives you answers. If it doesn't have answers, I direct you to some places where you can get them in the Appendix.

No matter what your level, this book can be a great addition to your library:

- ✔ As a novice, you can give yourself an introduction before you step foot in a class.
- ✔ As an intermediate practitioner, you can figure out the why behind something that you've been doing — and perhaps do it better.
- ✔ As an advanced student, you can read different takes and opinions about how to do a form that may broaden your world.

How to Use This Book

Have you ever been in a foreign country and had trouble reading store signs or package labels, despite having taken a foreign language for tourist class? What you needed was a quick and easy reference book so you could look up the sign and say, "Ah-ha, that's what that means!"

That's what this book is — a quick and easy reference guide that you can continually pick up, shuffle through, and go, "Ah-ha!" This book is also a simple introductory guide that allows you to answer a pressing question without the urgent ah-ha moment.

I don't think that this book should be the only T'ai Chi book on your shelf. Oh my, no. There are so many schools, styles, teachers, and traditions in T'ai Chi that you need an array of books to help you along your journey.

Imagine traveling in Europe: If you are spending a couple days in several countries, an all-encompassing European phrase book works just fine. But if you plan to spend a week or a month in one place, such as Spain, you need an entire Spanish phrase book for its detail.

The same thing goes for T'ai Chi. This is your all-encompassing phrase book — one that gives you a little bit about a lot of basic ideas. If you plan to spend more time in one area or develop an interest in one aspect, you need more-detailed specialty materials. So don't hesitate. I won't be insulted. In fact, I will be thrilled that you want to progress and that you felt tantalized enough by this book to want more.

In this book, I primarily write about T'ai Chi (pronounced tie-*jee*), although I touch on its close relative Qigong (chee-*gung*). I also introduce a few other kissing cousins, as well as a few sprinkles of philosophy and mind-body principles.

Basically though, I don't get deeply into the great philosophical roots of these mindful arts. This book is mostly about doing T'ai Chi — learning just enough so you can get up out of your chair and move a little.

When I introduce a movement that I expect you'll want to do, I also include pictures or illustrations, as necessary. Because T'ai Chi is all about flow, I refer back and forth between the written instruction and the illustrations to help you understand what is moving where and when. It's most helpful to your developing practice — and safer for you — if you read the instructions and review the illustrations first before getting up to try to movement yourself.

Try each movement alone first before you string a few together. Also, don't forget to review the basics in Chapter 8 before trying the forms in Chapters 9 through 12, because I refer back to those basics quite often.

Conventions Used in This Book

The illustrations are easy to read, moving left to right and top to bottom as most in the Western world. Occasionally I use arrows in the figures indicate the direction of movement of a limb. Remember, though, these are figures and not necessarily exact to the inch, because T'ai Chi's three dimensions aren't the easiest to portray on a flat page. Note, too, that the movements in the illustrations are done as if you were standing in one place and facing the person in the pictures as he or she begins the series of movements. This means that you'll look at the figure's side and back at times as they progress through the forms. This helps you constantly retain the correct perspective, because the forms turn throughout to face different directions.

Also, I often refer to someone named Manny. Manny Fuentes is my collaborator, a T'ai Chi instructor who has lent oodles of expertise, instruction, anecdotes, pieces of wisdom, and a great sense of humor to the book. To keep things simple, I (that's me — the writer, Therese Iknoian) am the only "I" in the book, and I just refer to Manny when something from him comes up. That way, you don't have two people to deal with calling themselves "I" (which may have made you wonder if I — Therese — had gone schizophrenic).

How This Book Is Organized

This book has six distinct parts, as well as an Appendix of resources that you don't want to miss. They are organized to help you best find your way along your T'ai Chi journey.

Part 1: Stepping Up to T'ai Chi

Before you set out on your T'ai Chi road, you want a map that gives you an overview of what you'll see along the way, as well as some introductory background not only on T'ai Chi, but also about mind-body movement. You see, T'ai Chi and mind-body theories are close-knit. This part is where you get some help setting your goals, find out about the health benefits, and get some definitions of basic terms that you see throughout the book.

Part II: Preparing to T'ai One On

Now I get more specific. This part gives you details about the history, traditions, and specific background of T'ai Chi. You get to pick apart some segments of practice, find out about how they relate, and perhaps most importantly, spend some time discovering some basic principles of the dance called T'ai Chi.

Part III: Knocking on T'ai Chi's Door

This part is where you find out about the movements, look at illustrations, and get up and move a little yourself. I break this section down by presenting the basics of foot, hand, and other techniques and transitions that come up later. Then I present the Yang Short Form. As an extra benefit, I also present a special shorter short form conceived by my collaborator Manny Fuentes, who is a long-time instructor. You can enjoy this brief form as a warm-up or as an addition to your regular T'ai Chi practice.

Part IV: Energizing Softly with Qigong

T'ai Chi and Qigong go together like salt and pepper. I would be remiss not to give you some basics about this meditative and chi-stimulating practice that is softer than even traditional T'ai Chi. So in this short part, you not only find out about the Qigong benefits, but you also find an introduction to some basic movements that you can do as a part of your practice.

Part V: Making the Most of Your Practice

This part discusses not only how you can practice T'ai Chi on your own but also how you can transfer the basics of the T'ai Chi principles to your daily life. You may be too busy to do an entire form or need some help deciding what to do, so I also put together some short combinations of movements presented earlier in this book, as well as a few other simple movements that make a nice addition to short practices.

Part VI: The Part of Tens

The Part of Tens presents fun, fast, flavorful facts in digestible and readable fashion. You find summaries of basic benefits, quick hints on how to supplement a practice, and some suggestions on where and when to practice. Plus, I give you two chapters with some great take-away pieces of wisdom and some thought-provoking quotes.

Icons Used in This Book

This little bulls-eye marks something that can help you better understand the current topic or gives you a pointer about something you can do.

These tidbits help you take note of an important fact because they point out why it's emphasized.

Watch out for these marks because they point out physical or mental precautions to keep you safe and help you progress.

This icon helps out in places where words or phrases can make you trip up.

T'ai Chi and Qigong are about flow and energy. So I make an effort to stress this point and give you ideas on how you can help incorporate more flow into your life. This is one of the more important icons!

Everybody has two cents to add, and I'm not any different. I use this icon to point out personal examples or experiences not only of mine but also of my collaborator, Manny. You find nifty stories and tales that can help you relate to T'ai Chi and that also serve to personalize the descriptions and instruction.

Taking on T'ai Chi should be enlightening, but it should also be fun. So look inside yourself, take the lessons and principles to heart, and don't forget to enjoy what you're doing, too.

Where Do I Go from Here?

When you reach for this book, use it as your whim strikes. If you're an orderly type who would never dream of reading the ending of a book first, feel free to start with Chapter 1 and read all the way through to the bits and pieces of information in the Appendix. If you're looking for an answer to a question or some snippet about a particular concept, check out the Table of Contents or the Index and then head straight for the chapter that you need.

Or, you can even just skip around as your fancy strikes, opening to a section of philosophy one day, history on another, movement the next, and maybe a Part of Tens chapter when you have only a few minutes to invest.

Heck, you can even fold down the corners of the pages, write little notes in the margins if you want, or circle particular figures on which you want to work. I do that to my books all the time. (The only problem with page-folding in my house is that I turn my page corners *away* from the page I'm referencing, and my husband turns them *toward* the page he's referencing. So we get confused all the time.)

You can also mark up the pictures if you find a different way to move a hand or foot as it works better for you. Re-draw them or doodle a little, if you will. Doodling isn't just for kindergartners.

It's all up to you at this point. Have fun!

Part I

Stepping Up to T'ai Chi

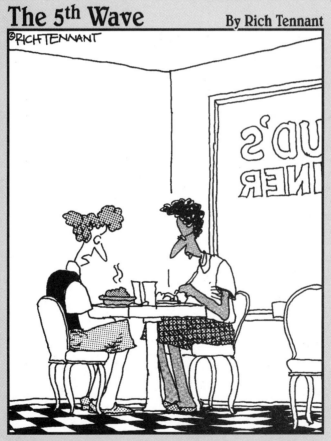

The 5th Wave   By Rich Tennant

"I'm always endeavoring to become one with all things, however I'm going to make an exception with this fish casserole."

In this part . . .

Your mindful journey is about to begin. Whether you've already dabbled in internal martial arts or you're simply intrigued, this part helps you lay the groundwork for a fulfilling and satisfying future T'ai Chi practice. In this part, you take a look at the reasons to practice T'ai Chi — as your only activity or as a supplement to other activities. You also get to peek into the scientific literature to find out what kind of benefits you may find through a T'ai Chi practice. Finally, you can discover the keys to harvesting true mind-body benefits. These keys are your first steps to knowing the important basics of T'ai Chi.

Chapter 1

Matching T'ai Chi's Mind-Body Benefits to Your Needs

Deciding to look into a T'ai Chi practice can be a pretty big step for many Westerners. If you want to exercise, you usually choose familiar stuff like riding a bike, walking, running, or swimming. These exercises are pretty straightforward in the Western world. You do the movements. You try not to think too hard about them. You huff and puff. You sweat. You may hurt a little the next day.

That's just the opposite of T'ai Chi. Sure you do the movements, but you don't huff and puff. You actually try to think about and focus on each move, using your mind — not just your body — as much as possible. T'ai Chi is soft and gentle. You may sweat, but just a little. And if you hurt the next day, you probably did too much or did something wrong.

Whoa, that can't be good for you, can it? Yes, it is good for you, whether you practice T'ai Chi by itself or as part of a routine that incorporates familiar movement forms like walking or swimming. (See Chapter 2 for details on T'ai Chi's benefits.)

But I jump ahead of myself. What is T'ai Chi, really?

Defining the Grand Ultimate

If you've picked up this book, you likely have some inkling about what T'ai Chi (properly pronounced tie-*jee,* but often heard as tie-*chee* in the West) is — or isn't. Or perhaps you aren't sure, and you're intrigued enough to shuffle through these pages.

Everybody was Kung Fu fighting...

And just so you can answer the trivia question at your next party, *Kung Fu* actually refers to the level of achievement earned by work over time.

It just so happens that in the West, we use it to mean Chinese martial arts.

Nevertheless, I start with the nitty-gritty. *T'ai Chi* is an ancient internal martial art — a mindful martial art — focusing on smooth, slow movements that cultivate inward focus and free energy flow. This type of martial art — compared to a non-mindful fighting art — wants you to use your mind to focus and move and, therefore, the "mindful" part. Some people even call T'ai Chi a *moving meditation.* T'ai Chi is rooted in the Taoist (pronounced *dow*-ist) philosophy of harmonious living. (You can find some great Taoist pieces of wisdom in Chapter 24.)

You may hear the term *mind-body fitness* to describe movement forms like T'ai Chi, as well as other stuff like yoga. That term is basically interchangeable with the descriptor *mindful* that I use. Although the definition of mindful movement is changing practically daily, one can loosely describe it as a "physical exercise executed with a profound inwardly directed focus." In other words, you use your muscles, but you also engage your mind. If you want more information on mind-body fitness, I've written an entire book on it: *Mind-Body Fitness For Dummies* (published by Hungry Minds, Inc.). It's all there.

T'ai Chi is a member of the martial arts family, just like all the other practices in which you engage in flamboyant, teeth-kicking combat. They all belong to the family called *Wushu,* which basically means "martial art" or traditional self-defense activities practiced with or without weapons. Other Wushu forms date back much further than T'ai Chi. Look closely at the movements that are part of the routines in this book (for example, the circling, torso-turning, hand-pushing, and leg lifting) to see the resemblance to fighting martial arts.

If you use your imagination to speed up the movements in Chapters 9 through 11 and pretend that a member of the Evil Empire is facing you, you can probably punch him in the stomach, knock him off his feet, or send him flying against a wall, a la "Wushu" style. Ouch!

But that's not why you practice T'ai Chi. Although some people practice T'ai Chi to perfect these movements (called *forms*), to gain inner strength, and to improve their combative martial arts, most people in the West practice T'ai Chi for the peace, inner calm, focus, energy, balance, stress relief, and body control.

Finding Out What's in a Name

I usually call this mindful martial art simply T'ai Chi, just as in the title of the book. But you need to know a little more about the name, the abbreviation, the translations, and the apostrophes that you may or may not see as you progress. The following sections explain what you need to know.

Abbreviations 'r' us

T'ai Chi is shorthand for T'ai Chi Chuan (tie-*jee*-chewon, said without dawdling over the "chew" then "won" but instead running the two syllables together quickly). For example, if your name is Susan Marie, everybody — except your mother — may call you Sue for short. But the West isn't the mother of T'ai Chi Chuan, so you can just call it T'ai Chi.

Parting from apostrophes

JARGON ALERT

Then you have the apostrophes that may look so odd to Western eyes when they're smack in the middle of a word. Some teachers and authors use *Tai Chi Chuan,* simply leaving out the curly squiggle. Or they shorten the name to *Tai Chi,* also opting to drop the apostrophe because it seems so foreign. I choose to leave off the *Chuan* but leave the apostrophe in *T'ai.* Still, that doesn't really matter.

Many authors and other experts vary in the use and placement of apostrophes in the words used here. You may see T'ai Chi Ch'uan, Tai Chi Ch'uan, and T'ai Chi Chuan — the last one being the one I use. Note the different apostrophe placements. You don't need to get wrapped up determining which style is right or wrong, or get hung up on phonetics and things, unless you want to delve into the ancient classical background and write your dissertation about this.

Throwing in another

T'ai Chi Ch'ih is a contemporary method that has some basis in the concepts of the ancient classical form of T'ai Chi Ch'uan's movement. Its movements are only reminiscent of T'ai Chi, based on the developer's own experience with it. This method has no true relation to T'ai Chi — except that it's slow and gentle.

Spelling: Not just for bees

You may also see T'ai Chi written as Taiji (tie-*jee*) or Taijiquan, which is more accurately Chinese but isn't commonly seen in the West. Same pronunciation, just more comfortable for the eyes because of the Latin letters.

Translation, please?

Now, about the translation of this T'ai Chi stuff. As with any foreign translation, you see a lot of variations. The name *T'ai Chi* can be translated from Chinese into English to mean something as simple as "The Grand Ultimate," "Great Extremes," "The High Peak," or "Superior Ultimate." Regardless, T'ai Chi means the incredibly important and unified really big thing.

Ch'uan simply means *fist*. Or you may see it used to mean *boxing* or some other kind of combative word. In this case, some may say the Chinese use *fist* to symbolize a complete embodiment.

So *T'ai Chi Ch'uan* is loosely translated as "The Grand Ultimate Fist" by some and "The Great Extremes" by others. You can choose which one to call it as you find out more. Does it really matter which name you use? A rose by any other name . . . Shakespeare was right.

Setting T'ai Chi Apart from Other Movements

One of the things that may seem strange about T'ai Chi is that you don't have to go harder, faster, or higher to reap fitness and health benefits. At first, T'ai Chi may feel and look unusual because its basic motto is contradictory to most familiar Western forms of exercise. (In China and other parts of Asia, T'ai Chi is mainstream, whereas fitness walking or jogging has been considered unusual, even odd, until recently.)

The T'ai Chi motto is the following: Go slow. Go slower. Go as slowly as you can. You may think that you are going as slowly as you can, but you aren't, so try to go slower. T'ai Chi is the complete opposite of hamsters-on-a-wheel step aerobics, hiking up a hill as fast as possible, or going as quickly as you can on the treadmill to burn more calories.

Always think slooooow, slooooower, slooooooowest. You are the tortoise, not the hare. Remember that fable? The tortoise wins the race.

In part, the slowness of T'ai Chi movements forces you to get in touch with your body, listen to your mind, and integrate them both until you're moving as one unified mass. When you do T'ai Chi, you can't let your brain plan tomorrow's dinner while your body goes through the motions.

Reasoning Your Way to T'ai Chi

Someone may want to dip his or her toes into T'ai Chi — or another meditative art, Qigong (see Chapters 13 and 14) — for several reasons. These reasons may be simple or complex, emotional or physical.

Fixating on fitness and exercise

Can something that looks like adults playing freeze tag be considered legitimate exercise? Ah, little Grasshopper, don't be so skeptical! Yes, T'ai Chi moves slowly, but take a quick glance at the summary of health benefits in Chapter 2 to ease any skepticism.

You may not get beefy biceps or be able to drop into Olympic gymnast splits, but not everyone needs that kind of fitness.

You can gain the following benefits from practicing T'ai Chi:

- **Aerobic fitness:** You can do T'ai Chi very slowly or you can pick up the tempo a bit as you become more advanced. You can keep the positions taller with straighter legs or you can bend your knees to challenge your muscles to make your heart and lungs work harder. Both are legitimate ways to move enough to raise your heart rate so that your heart and lungs become more fit and healthy.

- **Muscle strength:** Depending on your abilities, you can do T'ai Chi with nearly straight knees, which is easy on your leg and hip muscles, or you can do T'ai Chi squatted low to the ground to fully challenge all the muscles in your back, hips, buttocks, and legs. You may also find that holding your arms up against the force of gravity and moving them slowly but continuously can be more of an upper body workout than you ever dreamed.

- **Flexibility:** As you progress, you can challenge the flexibility of your entire body by, for example, lifting your legs higher in kicks, squatting lower and wider during moving forms, or stretching taller in arm movements or warm-ups.

Teetering over balance

Many people gravitate toward T'ai Chi because it improves their ability to balance. In other words, it keeps you from falling. Particularly seniors, and anybody who has weak ankles or weak lower legs, can gain better balance.

The improvements happen because of training better proprioception of the nerves and muscles in the lower legs. Loosely translated, *proprioception* is sort of like tickling the nerves and muscles to improve the muscle sense of the body's position in space. With better balance, you don't wobble as much or turn your ankles as often.

Rehabbing injuries and strains

It is perhaps a combination of both fitness and balance that allows T'ai Chi to be a great way to get stronger and pain-free after injuries or accidents. I practiced T'ai Chi following chronic ankle sprains to regain strength and to continue athletic training. My collaborator, Manny, originally got into T'ai Chi because of a back injury.

Minding your mind

Whether you are stressed out or just busy because of work, school, or family obligations, T'ai Chi gives you a chance to find an inner sea of calm.

You can't do T'ai Chi and stay stressed out. If you move slowly and breathe correctly, your stress dissipates, leaving you more relaxed and refreshed. Over time, you find out how to incorporate this stress release in daily life. For example, you can practice while stuck in a rush-hour traffic jam or standing in a long line at the bank behind someone who has 20 million checks to deposit and forgot to sign them. See Chapter 21 for tips on incorporating the principles of T'ai Chi into daily life.

Capturing the culture and tradition

A T'ai Chi practice isn't about only the physical and the mental exercises. You can also discover the cultural traditions and philosophies. Perhaps you're interested in finding out more about Taoist principles. These principles are ingrained in T'ai Chi practice, which is a great way to embrace them and make them a part of your life. Maybe you want to discover more about Chinese history and traditions. The history and traditions are studies in and of themselves, but for a glimpse look in Chapter 5. T'ai Chi is one avenue for finding out more about such traditions.

Finishing with Wise Words

As the saying goes, there are many paths to the mountain. The path that you choose to take may be a little different than the path another person chooses. But when you get to the top of the mountain, the view is the same.

Along the path, you may find that practicing T'ai Chi is a means to physical, mental, emotional, and spiritual elevation. The principles and practice of this ancient, internal martial art can permeate every aspect of your life — from your physical health and fitness to your view of the world and the way you interact with others around you. But, sigh, it can't happen overnight. Perhaps that's one of the reasons T'ai Chi has remained slightly esoteric as a regular practice in the United States. In the West, everybody seems to want things quickly — 2-minute abs, 5-minute dinners, and 10-minute oil changes.

When you start your practice, one thing that you need to learn is patience. Manny says that in nearly every class he starts, someone pops up a hand and asks, "How long will it take me to learn T'ai Chi?" Manny says that he stops, ponders the question quietly, and then usually answers, "I don't know. As soon as I feel that I've learned it, I'll let you know."

You see, T'ai Chi is a lifelong learning. You're never truly done. Think of Einstein's comment that the larger the circle of knowledge becomes, the larger the circumference of darkness is. In other words, the more you know, the more you realize that you still have to learn. Anyone who says that he or she is a T'ai Chi expert is stomping all over one of the basic Taoist credos of humility, which is to recognize that you never know it all. Even masters are still learning. Don't set arbitrary time constraints for your learning. Attainment in T'ai Chi is measured in years or even lifetimes, not weeks or days

As you dive into T'ai Chi, all you need to do for success in your practice is the following:

1. **Start.**

2. **Continue.**

That's all folks. Just remember, the journey of a thousand miles begins with one single step. So journey forth. Find peace and calm, and let the journey itself be your goal.

Chapter 2

Evaluating T'ai Chi's Health Benefits with a Western Mind

*W*estern scientific minds have managed to put their stamp of approval on the basics of fitness and health — what to do, how much to do, and how hard to do it. Although their guidelines can change year to year, the basics remain about how you can stay in the best health using activity and movement. Then, heck, here comes this Eastern stuff about movement types and methods that doesn't exactly jibe with Western wisdom about what you *should* do. And that confuses the protocol-driven researchers in the West.

Before you fully dive into your T'ai Chi practice, you need to know a little bit about beliefs and theories on both sides. Then you can decide how you want to mix and match them into your own practice and what works best for you. As always, caution is the first stepping stone.

Prepping for a Safe, Sane Practice

If you plan to do high kicks, pump up your heart rate, or crank out tough calisthenics — and if these exercises are all new to you — you need to take into account your current health before moving ahead. That includes seeing a physician for clearance, particularly if you're older than 40.

But even the gentlest of movements, such as T'ai Chi or Qigong (another mindful Asian movement art that I discuss in more depth in Chapters 13 and 14), can put uncommon strains on your muscles, back, joints, or heart from bending, twisting, holding, or squatting movements. So to be on the safe side, lay a solid and sane groundwork to make sure that your journey is wise, healthful, and fruitful. I encourage you take the following questionnaire seriously.

If you answer "yes" to any of the following questions, see a physician before starting an exercise program.

If you don't answer "yes" to any of these questions, but you are age 40 or older or you haven't exercised regularly in a year or more, you should still see a physician to check on your overall health and to discuss any medical conditions that may run in your family.

Don't let any of these warnings scare you off from movement! It simply makes good sense to see a physician once a year anyway. If at any time an answer to one of the questions changes to "yes" during your exercise program, you need to check with your physician.

- ✔ Are you currently not exercising regularly?
- ✔ Do you have a personal or family history of heart disease or chest pains, especially before age 50?
- ✔ Do you smoke or have you been a smoker in the past two years?
- ✔ Do you have any joint problems, such as achiness or stiffness, that get worse when you move in certain ways?
- ✔ Do you have high blood pressure, diabetes, high cholesterol, or high blood sugar?
- ✔ Are you taking any medications for any of the preceding conditions that may change the way your body responds to exercise?
- ✔ Are you considered very overweight or obese? (I'm not talking about an extra 10 to 20 pounds here.)
- ✔ Do you know of any other reason why you should not do physical activity?

Going West for Eastern Movement

Perhaps you know the basics of what the scientific and exercise gurus say that you need to do for good health and fitness. They call it an "exercise prescription," which never sounded too palatable to me. Isn't a prescription something like bad-tasting cough syrup? Nevertheless, the federal Centers for Disease Control and Prevention, the American Heart Association, and the American College of Sports Medicine have come up with guidelines, which I present in this section.

Although the "traditional" Western way of exercise isn't necessarily applicable to Eastern movement like T'ai Chi, the "less traditional" way, as defined in the West, can be. And it doesn't hurt to see how your chosen path fits in with the following guidelines.

Speaking aerobically

Aerobic exercise is activity that raises your heart rate. T'ai Chi and Qigong — depending on the style you choose and the tempo you pick — can actually raise your heart rate from a small amount to a moderate amount, although that really isn't your goal.

Going the traditional way

The traditional Western exercise model is the recognizable way to improve aerobic fitness, lose weight, or achieve better physical performance. I'm not talking mindful meditation here. For that, you can turn to Chapter 4 where you can read more about the keys to reaping mind-body benefits.

The traditional regimen requires activity:

- 3 to 5 days a week

- For 20 to 60 minutes at a time

- At 60 to 90 percent of maximum heart rate (or at an effort that is moderate to pretty hard). That's equal to about 4 to 9 on a scale of 0 to 10 where 0 is doing nothing and 10 is all-out. For more information on figuring your maximum heart rate, see the nearby sidebar, "Taking it to the max: Your heart rate."

Taking a less traditional approach

In 1995, the exercise gurus came up with a less formal approach to movement that can still get you healthy. It's a softer approach, much like Eastern mindful arts. The difference, however, is that you chose T'ai Chi for a distinct and internal purpose. This softer recommendation for activity was developed partly because most of the Western population couldn't get its act together to do the traditional method.

The beauty of this method is that it acknowledges lighter forms of activity, such as T'ai Chi or Qigong (Chapters 13 and 14 give you details about what Qigong is and how to do it).

The less traditional approach asks for movement:

- On most days

- For 30 minutes at a time

- At light to moderate intensity, where you feel you're moving at an effort that feels somewhere between 1-6 on a scale of 0-10 where 0 is lazing on the couch and 10 is going as hard as you can.

Taking it to the max: Your heart rate

Many mind-body methods, including T'ai Chi and Qigong, are based on the benefits you reap from being mindful and focused. These methods are generally more focused on a sense of effort, making your heart rate not as telling — or as necessary — as how you feel.

But if you choose more highly aerobic forms of T'ai Chi or Qigong (or forms that can become more aerobic), taking your heart rate can prove beneficial, especially if you wear a wireless heart rate monitor so you don't have to stop and put two fingers on your wrist and count (an activity that can really interrupt your flow). Your physician may also advise taking your heart rate to help you maintain appropriate intensity.

So, how do you know what heart rate is right for you? The simplest way (although the number is truly a rough estimate) is to take your age and subtract it from 226 for women, 220 for men. That number is your maximum heart rate. Now, multiply it by the desired target percentage (which the next paragraph can help you determine) to get your target heart rate. If you are under a physician's care, he or she can advise you about the best percentage.

A low-intensity workout should raise your heart rate to less than about 55 to 60 percent of your maximum heart rate. A moderate workout raises it to about 60 to 75 percent, depending on your fitness level. A vigorous workout is anything about that, again depending on your fitness level (and vigorous workouts are in fact not truly advised to achieve mindful benefits). Most beneficial mind-body routines fall between about 55 and 70 percent of maximum heart rate.

For example, a 40-year-old woman has a maximum heart rate of 186. She wants to work our moderately, or at about 70 percent of her maximum. She multiplies .70 times 186 for a result of 130. Her target heart rate therefore is approximately 130, if she chooses to use heart rate as a way to measure her effort.

Know that you can have a margin of error of up to 10 to 15 beats in either direction using this estimate. So using a number that corresponds to your sense of effort can be very helpful and perhaps better for most mind-body methods. To find stories about heart rate as well as a heart rate calculator (to make your life easier), go to www.totalfitnessnetwork.com, where you can find a whole section on this subject, written by yours truly.

Getting a grip on strength

Strength-building movement also offers traditional and less-than-traditional approaches. Although not necessarily an intended result, the less traditional approach recognizes such movement as T'ai Chi as a way to keep muscles stronger.

Going the traditional way

The traditional Western idea is to increase your muscle strength and endurance with the following regimented workout pattern:

✔ 2 to 3 days a week

✔ 8 to 10 muscle groups each time (for example, the back, the chest, or the thighs)

✔ 8 to 12 repetitions per muscle group (A *repetition* is the number of times you do an exercise before resting.)

✔ 1 to 3 sets of repetitions (A set is the number of groups of repetitions you do.)

The traditional way can translate into spending too much time in a sweaty gym.

Taking a less traditional approach

In 2000, following a huge review of all the research, the exercise gurus found that you don't have to do quite as much or be as structured as in the traditional approach to improve your overall health.

The new statement called for a routine — still a bit regimented — that includes the following:

✔ 2 to 3 days a week

✔ 8 to 10 muscle groups each time

✔ 8 to 10 repetitions per muscle group

✔ 1 set (only one!) of repetitions

You may wonder how this approach applies to the mindful martial arts in this book. Well, you indeed use many muscle groups in a light way during your T'ai Chi forms. These muscle groups not only include your feet, lower legs, upper legs, hips, and buttocks, but also your back, chest, and arms.

Although you aren't doing sets of, say, bench presses or squats with plates of iron, you may be surprised at the strength you can gain. Still, because we in the West don't live the strenuous daily lives of yore, most experts advise adding a bit of strength-training, even to your program of mindful Asian movement arts, for really well-rounded and functional strength.

Knowing What Western Science Says about Eastern Movement

If you're a left-brained, show-me-the-proof kind of person, you may not particularly like what comes next: Researchers haven't turned out enough quality, air-tight, peer-reviewed, placebo-controlled, statistically significant scientific studies to make the kind of wonderful conclusions that you and I may want to make — and that some practitioners indeed do make.

Reviewing the reviews

A review of scientific literature published in early 2000 found "a dearth of randomized controlled research conducted in the U.S." The Stanford University authors, who had done an extensive search of most literature since 1990 and some before, went on to say that mind-body methods — including T'ai Chi and Qigong — seemed to be a great way to complement traditional treatments, but "most apparent was the need for further controlled research." I love this great big "out" in research — you just get to say "more research is needed."

Now, should you snap shut this book, slide it up on the highest shelf, and walk away? Heck no! Did you decide to read about or do some T'ai Chi because the experts say that it is good for you? I doubt it. It would be nice if everybody agreed that T'ai Chi and other Chinese mindful movement can be the one practice that alone will make you strong as an ox and even help you win the New York Marathon. But do they need to agree? No.

Don't get the researchers wrong. They aren't ogres. Many researchers would love to come up with a truly airtight way to say, "By Jove, I've got it!" But for methods like T'ai Chi, finding a truly scientific and air-tight way to present a study in which the subjects don't know what the goal is can be very difficult to achieve. If subjects know a study's hypothesis, the results can be tainted. Human nature wants to please, so subjects can actually talk themselves into believing that something happened, or they may just say that it happened to make a researcher happy. For example, "Am I less stressed after that class? Well, uh, why yes! Of course I am!" That doesn't make for any news that you can use.

Sleuthing out the claims

The only problem is, not having 100-perent airtight studies leaves a plethora of curative claims — some less than reputable, and some purely anecdotal but perhaps not so far-fetched — through which you must search and choose to believe, or search and destroy.

One scientific note: The United States government has now recognized mindful and alternative practices. The National Institutes of Health has a branch called the National Center for Complementary and Alternative Medicine (take a look at the appendix for how to find it). Its goal is to spark and fund research in these areas. So who knows what kind of great science will be discovered five or ten years down the road?

The power of the mind

Perhaps you've heard of the *placebo effect*, in which a harmless, unmedicated substance is used as a control in testing the effects of another substance or situation. For example, the effect comes into play when researchers give patients a sugar pill and tell them it will make them sleep better. If the mind overpowers the body, the people indeed sleep better. The same idea applies with mindful movement: You join a Qigong class because you hear it relieves arthritis pain; several weeks later, you indeed have less pain. You begin taking T'ai Chi because you've read that doing so will lower your blood pressure; a few weeks later — voila! — you have lower blood pressure.

Thus, the $60 million question: Is the possibility that the placebo effect occurred a bad thing? Well, if you practice T'ai Chi and become fitter, healthier, or pain- or disease-free, you didn't do yourself any harm. The mind has been shown to have a powerful effect on the body, whether spiritually or just hopefully. Meditative and mindful movement takes this power and actively applies it. So whether you believe in the mindful benefit, the spiritual benefit, the healing energy pulsing through the body, or, well, you just believe, you may indeed find what you want or need.

So for now, if you hear or read some health claims or tales of sudden cures, take them in with an open but analytical mind, and don't fall hook, line, and sinker. They may not be bogus, but they may need a more in-depth look.

In the next section, I cite a few claims — some taken from reputable studies, and some from less reputable studies but still worth peeking at. Either way, they are food for thought, like the anecdotes you hear of disappearing diseases and evaporating pains. Who am I to argue with my first T'ai Chi teacher, who described how he started practicing when he was diagnosed with a brain tumor about four decades ago? Now, there is no sign of any tumor. This kind of hearsay about T'ai Chi practice can mean more to you than some laboratory research done by planting electrodes on someone's body.

None of this information should make you dump your doc and try something like curing liver cancer through meditation. Instead, consult with your doctor to see whether a practice like T'ai Chi is appropriate for you. Perhaps supplementing your traditional medical care with some nontraditional Chinese moving meditation may help you feel better. Read on to see what areas T'ai Chi has been found to be the most helpful.

Science will probably never have all the answers when it comes to movement like T'ai Chi. But even the most perfect study may not give you better balance, make you more relaxed, and help you reduce stress, too.

Making the Benefits Work for You

Now I take a gander through the scientific literature. And you can come along, too. Some benefits are proven. Some are not but are interesting nonetheless. (See the section "Knowing What Western Science Says about Eastern Movement," earlier in this chapter.) In this section, you get a good look at the physical and mental benefits of T'ai Chi and Qigong.

The following information isn't a thorough and exacting scientific review. Instead, you get a pleasant tour, where I share a few scientific sites with you.

Betting on the benefits

T'ai Chi and Qigong — both mindful and meditative movement arts — may give you the best physical and mental benefits, depending on how much, at what intensity, with what seriousness, and how often you incorporate them into your life.

But you got me on this one: Maybe you can't really bet on these benefits, because some of them aren't completely proven by fully recognized scientific studies (see the section "Knowing What Western Science Says about Eastern Movement," earlier in this chapter). Of the studies that have been done, some haven't excluded bias by subjects or researchers, and some studies haven't been *replicated,* which means that the results haven't been repeated. (Replication is key for scientists, because they can determine that the results didn't occur by chance. In other words, they can verify a conclusion because the same thing happens again.)

Nonetheless, the variety benefits may include the following. For more details, take a look at Chapter 20:

- Better cholesterol levels
- Decreased depression
- Decreased risk of cardiovascular disease
- Increased immunity (less sickness)
- Increased muscle strength and flexibility
- Less lower back pain
- Less asthma

Now, that's quite a laundry list of possible health benefits! Don't forget that many of these perks — or to what extent you reap them — depend on the type or intensity of movement you choose.

Balancing your act

Good balance has been easier to study than some other areas. And T'ai Chi develops this skill well.

The physical balance that you can hone through the movements in T'ai Chi and Qigong can train the *proprioception* of the nerves and muscles (basically, the muscle sense). When the muscles and nerves can sense correctly how and when to contract or fire, you don't fall or get hurt. Staying upright can help decrease not only sports injuries but also broken hips in seniors, especially if a senior's bones are affected by bone-weakening osteoporosis.

Staying upright

Broken hips and other bones caused when seniors fall can cost the health care system heaps of money. But more importantly, the injuries can cause these seniors mountains of despair because they can lose some of their independence. Maintaining strong bones that can withstand a bump here and there is vital, and being able to stay upright can mean the difference between living in a nursing home or in your own home.

One 1997 study had senior subjects report back to researchers four months after completing 15 weeks of T'ai Chi training, simple balance training, education about exercise, or nothing. The subjects who had T'ai Chi or balance training said that they were more confident about daily movement, but only T'ai Chi subjects said their overall life and sense of well-being had improved.

Preserving core strength

T'ai Chi's emphasis on slow, flowing movements mandates abdominal strength and one-legged balance throughout the practice. You may not actually hold a stance for a long time, but you move through it. To achieve the smooth flow of T'ai Chi, you must have balance and torso strength, perhaps more so than to perform more traditional calisthenics.

Rehabilitating injuries

Balance is about more than not breaking hips. It's also about high-powered running performance or backpacking and hiking on narrow and rocky trails. These two activities can result in sprained ankles or even lower back pain.

Develop better balance and muscle sense, and you may become a better or more confident athlete after the injury is gone.

Stamping out bad or excess stress

It's one thing to say, "I feel less stress." That's something that anybody can appreciate. But it's another thing to see results of less stress, such as a decrease in heart disease.

Lowering your stress and anxiety

A slow and prolonged *exhalation* (the breathing out part of breathing) has been shown to enhance a reaction in the body that causes overall muscular relaxation. If you are more relaxed, you handle your stress and your emotions more easily, and you may even sleep better.

One study specifically compared moving T'ai Chi practices to walking and found that reactions in the body during T'ai Chi were similar to the reactions caused by moderate fitness walking in reducing anxiety and increasing vigor. Of course, researchers pointed out that people may have been biased after hearing about the wonderful relaxing effects of T'ai Chi. But is that such a terrible thing?

Subjects in other studies have reported less depression, anxiety, confusion, and tension in addition to an overall better mood.

Another study, reported in 1996 out of Korea, showed that Qigong training reduced certain hormones in the blood caused by stress. The claim is that Qigong is a way to cope with stress.

Lowering your risk of heart disease

When you aren't bound up by stress and anxiety, you feel better on a day-to-day basis. But living without stress and anger may also lower your blood pressure, lower your bad cholesterol level, and cause decreases in other factors that can raise your risk of heart disease.

One recent journal article reviewed research about meditation and relaxation techniques (although not specifically mind-body exercise) and found a reduced risk of coronary artery disease. Harvard physician Herbert Benson, who coined the term "relaxation response," says that changes with simple meditation, including lower blood pressure, can be achieved with such practices as T'ai Chi. Yet another article, which also looked at such areas as relaxation breathing, found fewer secondary heart attacks after five years of treatment in patients with heart disease.

Because of their slow and gentle ways, T'ai Chi practices have also been used successfully in cardiac rehabilitation programs.

Managing chronic disease

Chronic disease can mean any number of medical conditions, such as diabetes, *hypertension* (high blood pressure), arthritis, *fibromyalgia* (a muscle disease that causes ongoing pain), or just chronic pain.

Coping with high cholesterol or high blood pressure

Many studies have compared results from three groups: one that did meditative Qigong walking, one that did regular walking, and one that did nothing. The group that did Qigong walking, which is so slow that it doesn't really raise your heart rate to the level of any kind of aerobic workout, still ended up with lower resting heart rates. A lower resting heart rate can mean a stronger heart, and a stronger heart can mean fewer problems with cholesterol and blood pressure.

Combating asthma or breathing disorders

Enter the positive effects of breathing. Practicing full and deep breathing can stimulate the lungs and can cause positive increases in the amount of air you can get into and out of your lungs. If you can get more air in and more air out, you may be able to diminish the effects of asthma or other breathing ailments.

Relieving arthritis and other chronic pain

People with arthritis or other kinds of joint pain know that every move can hurt, so they tend to move less. And the reduced movement causes the muscles and tendons that support their joints to get very weak.

Over the years, studies have shown that simple, gentle movements help relieve arthritis and other chronic pain and allow people with these ailments to function better day-to-day. T'ai Chi and Qigong have been used as the gentle movement needed to stimulate the joints and free up movement to relieve pain. This same kind of movement may help alleviate pain. I'm talking about chronic pain, which can confound doctors if they can't determine the source. Sometimes, the pain is diffuse and can't be pinpointed. But over the years, many studies have shown that gentle and low-intensity movement relieves such pain.

One of many hundreds of studies done in China required two groups of pain patients to take Qigong classes. One class studied with a *master,* someone who is able to "move energy" and heal with his or her energy. The other class was led by a *sham master,* someone who can do the movements but isn't considered a healer. Pain decreased in both groups, although researchers think that happened because participants just believed in the practice. But pain symptoms in the group with the master went down twice as much!

Fostering fitness

Maybe T'ai Chi isn't just about preventing broken hips or blood pressure. Maybe T'ai Chi is also about complementing your overall fitness — balancing muscles, strengthening them, helping them become more flexible, or helping your heart and lungs develop more aerobic capacity. Maybe you want to finish a marathon or ride a bike better up hills. Even the gentle movements involved in T'ai Chi can help.

Perhaps T'ai Chi is about increasing strength and flexibility so you can get in and out of chairs more easily or up and down stairs.

Mastering muscle strength and flexibility

For someone old or young who is very out of shape, the gentle movements of T'ai Chi can push muscles to get stronger and more flexible. Of course, if you push your forms a bit faster, make the squatting movements lower, or make the kicks higher, you can improve your muscles and flexibility even more — perhaps as much as with some traditional exercise. Some studies in Asia have shown more flexibility and strength as a result of a T'ai Chi practice.

Even if science hasn't totally proven this idea, I suggest that you try T'ai Chi and see how you feel. My bet is you'll be surprised what something so seemingly gentle can do for you.

Then there's stretching for flexibility — something that most people don't do enough of and may find tedious. Something about the static from holding different positions can cause ants in your pants. T'ai Chi, on the other hand, can result in flexibility through more dynamic reaches and stretches.

Increasing aerobic endurance

Think that these slow-moving forms don't give you the aerobic pump that you need or want? Think again. Even a slow but steady class that is sequenced and paced appropriately can produce moderate increases in aerobic ability, or about half to two-thirds the benefits of traditional aerobic programs, such as running or group exercise. That's not small potatoes for something so simple.

Chapter 3

Building the Mind-Body Foundation

T'ai Chi is all about benefits to the mind *and* the body. So if you're a newcomer to mind-body movement of any kind — say, you've never even done something like Yoga — you may want to take a look at some basics before you forge ahead. These concepts are important to know in some way so that you can move on to T'ai Chi with a better base of knowledge.

Practicing T'ai Chi is like building a house. First, you have to build the mindful foundation — the tenets in this chapter. Next you can start putting up the framework — the basis of the principles and parts of T'ai Chi practice (see Chapters 7 and 8). Then, and only then, can you safely and securely add the roof and the walls — which are the movements and the forms (see Chapters 9 through 11).

You can decorate your house by deepening your practice and truly immersing yourself in the more-advanced forms of practice — and the philosophy, some of which is introduced in Chapter 6. But you add these decorations after you build your T'ai Chi house (just as putting flowers on the windowsill or shutters on the window isn't the first thing you do).

You may hear about other mind-body theories and concepts from different practitioners and teachers. Good! I won't tell you that the principles and tenets presented in this book as the foundation are the only ones. Or that the way presented in this book is the only way to break down those principles and basics as you progress. There are a million (okay, I exaggerate a little) different ways to slice a cake. So enjoy this slice. And next time you can enjoy another slice!

While you enjoy the slice presented in this book, you can begin by looking at a mindful foundation that is the first step toward T'ai Chi's foundation. I split this foundation — remember how you build your house in the preceding paragraphs — into five areas:

- ✔ **Breath:** Full, deep, conscious, and grounded
- ✔ **Relaxation:** Loose and without stress for even more power
- ✔ **Alignment:** Relaxed, yet strong, and rooted firmly to the ground, while sensing nearly a suspension from above
- ✔ **Visualization:** Using your mind for your purpose, with control
- ✔ **Energy:** Connecting to your energy, others' energy, and the earth's energy

Want more? Then read on as I go a little deeper into each area in the next section.

Breathing Fully and Easily

Breath is life. Breath is energy. You can live for weeks without food and for days without water, but only for minutes without breathing the air in and out of your body. Breathing not only keeps you alive, but it also gives you more energy and more calm so you can face what life brings you. That's why breathing is so vital.

Manny tells a story about his friend who is a singer and songwriter. As a fledgling songwriter himself, Manny says that he once asked his friend for a couple of pointers about singing. His friend replied, "It's all about air." Well, that's the same advice — albeit basic — that I give you about a good T'ai Chi practice.

The problem is that most people don't pay attention to their breathing. What? As if I have to pay attention to my breath? Breathing isn't like driving a car, where you have to think about putting your foot on the brake to stop. Or so you think, right?

Breathing just happens. But does good, healthful, and mindful breathing just happen? The answer, in most cases, is no. For most of us, the involuntary, subconscious breathing we do is shallow, weak, and not necessarily timed to anything except our bodies demand to suck in more air to survive. Conscious breathing, as needed here, is a breath that comes with particular movements, or in particular moments, and is deeper and more energizing. For more, read on.

Keeping the air going in and out

The first part of breathing is the simple process of keeping air going in and out of your system for more success, safety, and comfort.

If you've ever taken a group exercise class, you probably remember the instructor constantly saying, "Breathe!" Perhaps you've heard it so much that you tune it out.

Now's the time not only to tune in that voice, but to make it your own. One simple, focused, well-timed breath can mean success in many movements, not to mention in daily life.

Fully tapping into the energy and calm

The next part of breathing is *conscious breathing:* Using the breath for the successful management and direction of energy in your body. But this means a full and deep breath, not a little, shallow, tight wheeze.

A full *inhalation* (that's when you breathe in) moves all the way down your abdomen and inflates your belly a little without causing your chest or shoulders to move upward much at all. If you're like many people, the breaths you take make your chest and ribs puff upward and then just stop without moving down into the belly. Try inhaling again, letting the inhalation move your belly out.

Attentive breathing is a remarkably effective way to clear and relax your mind. Tune into yourself whenever you start to feel a little stressed or tense. I lay money down that you find yourself holding your breath or breathing very tightly and highly in your chest. I do! As I work along, I have made it a conscious part of my time to take conscious breaths. They just feel so good!

Practicing the right way

Then you have the matter of the right way to breathe. With T'ai Chi, things are pretty simple compared to other mindful methods that advocate breathing with different rhythms or using your nose and/or your mouth. I get into the specific breathing principles of T'ai Chi in Chapter 7.

For now, remember that breathing with movement helps you with movement — even if the movement is just standing up from your chair! Usually, you *exhale* — or breathe out — when you are exerting energy during a movement like pushing your hand forward, and you *inhale* — or breathe in — when you are relaxing or retreating, such as pulling a hand back. Note the contrast to how breath is used in daily life: One big exhale is often considered relaxing, but that's usually when you aren't doing anything.

I can state the three main concepts about breathing pretty darn simply:

 ✔ Breathe consciously.

 ✔ Breathe fully.

 ✔ Breathe with the movement.

Relaxing the Muscles

The power in everything you do doesn't come from intense muscular effort but from muscular relaxation. When the body is properly aligned and relaxed, you can conjure up an amazing amount of power with seemingly little effort. Whether it's ballet, hammering a nail, or practicing T'ai Chi, beginners almost always try too hard to get it right too soon. Been there? Yeah, I thought so. Me too.

Funny thing is, if you relax and use the body's inner strength, you can get it right faster.

I'm not talking about floppy-fish body relaxation. Following are two ways to use your muscles, and I'm talking about using one of them. (Hint: the *second* one.)

 ✔ **Gripping:** Muscle use often accompanied by clenched teeth, a clamped jaw, or clenched, white-knuckled fingers. Not to mention all the surrounding muscles that get tight even when they don't need to. This builds tension and usually stops a conscious breath. (See the section, "Breathing Fully and Easily," earlier in this chapter.)

 ✔ **Contracting:** Using a specific muscle for movement, without involving any muscles not required for the movement — including that nasty ol' clenched jaw. This method usually allows relaxation and continuous full and deep breathing to accomplish the movement well.

Experiment with me for a moment to see what you do:

 1. **Raise one arm up in front of you from your shoulder.**

 2. **Now tighten your shoulder muscle.**

Is your fist clenched and your bicep bundled up? Hold on. You should tighten your *shoulder,* not the entire arm. Now, try again: Keep the shoulder tightened while you relax your bicep, forearm, and fingers. (Don't forget to keep your jaw relaxed.) Feels different that way, doesn't it? You're probably still breathing, too.

Opposites attract: Yin and yang

Life is about opposites — salt and pepper, black and white, hot and cold, hard and soft, love and hate, light and dark. The law of opposites also applies to mind-body movements — forward and back, *full* (weight-bearing) and *empty* (non-weight-bearing), high and low, reach and pull back.

These balancing moves are opposing yet complementary, and they highlight the ancient Chinese philosophy of yin and yang, which are basically placeholders for opposites. (See the accompanying figure.) *Yin* has more to do with softness and receptivity, a more emotional energy, and often includes movements that are lower (of the earth). *Yang* has more to do with hardness and creativity, a more muscular energy, and includes movements that are higher (representative of the sky).

No movement is actually purely one or the other, yin or yang, because one part manifests yang as another part manifests yin. You are constantly shifting and moving between the two.

In Chinese philosophy, yin represents the feminine nature of the universe, and yang represents

the masculine. T'ai Chi tries to keep you balanced between the yin and yang of movement, creating a flowing and rhythmical dance between the two. Applying this philosophy in everyday life can have benefits, too. The yin-yang symbol shown in the figure is perfectly symmetrical. The symbol doesn't have any angles or places where energy stops or pools, and one side isn't better or larger than the other. The yin and yang flow together and accept each other because both are necessary to everything that is life.

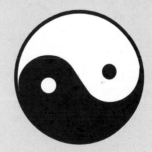

Have you ever floated on your back in water? If you fight the water by flailing and splashing, you can't begin to float. But if you relax and breathe, you can float effortlessly — even though you're using some muscular contraction. To build a better mind-body foundation, all you need to do is float effortlessly, using only the muscles needed.

Aligning and Rooting Your Body

Alignment and posture aren't about your legs. They're about your *core,* your center, the lower part of your torso. (You may call it your abs, but a good-centered alignment goes deeper than superficial abdominal muscles.)

Your physical *power center* is right in your core. This area is basically around your belly button and abdominals. With a strong core, you can accomplish a well-rooted alignment that is connected from head to toe. (I'm not talking six-pack abs, mind you. Again, that's too superficial.)

If you try to walk, balance, stand up from sitting, reach into a cabinet, or do any kind of common sports or daily movement without your core engaged, you aren't able to move smoothly, strongly, or with any amount of control. No matter what you do, imagine that the movement resonates from your power center and not from the limb doing the action.

A strong core can't be strong if you kind of hang over it. I discuss the basics of T'ai Chi posture in Chapter 8, which is a good place to go for more details on T'ai Chi. In Chapter 13, you can find a short discussion on the energy points in the body and how they relate to your core.

Meanwhile, think that you are strong "to the core." Ever wonder why people say that something is good or bad to the core? Because the core is the center of what you're all about.

Dancers and other movement artists use the core's power and the strong alignment of the body to allow them to perform sensational feats, such as leaping across a stage looking as though they are hanging from a wire, or even balancing on a high wire! Mindfully speaking, your core is the fountain of all your body's energy, and according to the theories of some mind-body practices, the core must be worked and massaged so you can break free of pain, fill yourself with positive energy, successfully complete a move, or find the true meaning of bliss.

Visualizing and Using Your Mind

Mind-body practices can't exist without the mind. You say, "No kidding, Sherlock." That's settled, then. I'm glad that you and I agree with all the Chinese internal martial art philosophers.

Using your mind means using it — not just letting it go along for the ride — to see not only what you're going to do, but sort of *inside* what you're going to do. When you start to perform any action in T'ai Chi, you *visualize* it. In other words, you think it through first. You see yourself completing it. You imagine the energy flowing to all the right places. You know that you're relaxed, not tense. And you can even visualize the breath moving in and out and through your body.

Look at it this way

When you start doing some mindful movements in T'ai Chi or Qigong, you may not be sure where to look with your eyes. Your eyes may sort of skip furtively about, catching some dust that you should wipe up on a shelf, something on the floor that you should put away, or a neighbor in the yard next door.

Wandering eyes distract you from putting T'ai Chi concepts into full practice. You need to see — without truly seeing. Here's a tip: Soften your gaze as if your eyes are open but nobody's home. You want to look inward and focus on your breath and relaxation. Let the gaze follow your fingertips, although you aren't really looking at them. The eyeballs are just moving in the same direction. You can also try some movements with your eyes closed, but work into keeping them open or halfway open.

Visualizing connects many of the concepts in this chapter. Because visualizing is not just about relaxing, breathing, and aligning. It's about *seeing* it. And visualizing is not just about mechanically doing something the way that you are told. It's about *feeling* it.

In the practice of *Hsing-I,* otherwise known as "mind-shape boxing," the mind forms the intent, and the body follows. The mental aspects make internal martial arts, such as T'ai Chi, more than just ways to use the body. They become platforms for the discovery and elevation of your character.

Jim Lau, a well-known instructor of a martial art called Wing-Chun, has said: "I can defeat you physically with or without a reason. But I can only defeat your mind with a reason."

Use your mind, and the body will follow.

Finding Energy Central

Ever turn on the hose to water your garden or lawn, only to have a mere trickle of water dribble out? Chances are, the first thing you did was size up the length of the hose for a twist or a kink. Like a kinked water hose, a body that isn't aligned, relaxed, breathing, and visualizing can't let its energy flow smoothly and efficiently. And the body can't soak up the energy around it or in the earth or trees, or apply any of that energy for its benefit.

Mind-body movements rely on a good and full energy flow. But even non-mindful movements require the power that comes with a surge of focused energy!

If you think that this energy stuff seems esoteric, you can find more about energy and its points of access in Chapter 13.

In mind-body arts, energy is described many ways, from simply energy and *chi* (which translates loosely to "life energy" in the Chinese forms) to power, intrinsic energy, vital life force, breath of life, and so on. I call it *energy* or *chi* (pronounced *chee*). Note that you may also see chi spelled as *qi,* as in Qigong, another mindful movement art I introduce in Chapters 13 and 14. Both are acceptable, although some practitioners lean more toward one or the other. But don't let that confuse you. Whether you say *chi* or *qi,* it's the same thing.

All the descriptions of energy mean the same thing, no matter how esoteric or concrete the term: Everybody is born to this Earth with a life force or energy central in their core within their body. Many people block the energy because of cultural or physical reasons.

Feeling the energy flow can be an emotional and even a healing experience, perhaps even scary. (I lead you through some ways to feel your energy in Chapter 14.) But nurturing a full and unkinked flow of chi is the goal of all mind-body movement, particularly T'ai Chi and Qigong. Without a free internal chi flow, these forms are not *mind*-body movement, but simply *body* movement. Now, if all you want is a little gentle exercise, forget this chi stuff. But if you want to gain more benefits in the long-term, think about and work on connecting to the earth, to yourself, to others, to the heavens, and on feeling yourself flow. And that can only be achieved by applying all the concepts in this chapter.

In this book, I don't go into huge philosophical depth about chi and the energy channels (see Chapter 13) through which energy flows in your body. If you want more information, refer to the Appendix for resources to further your journey.

For now, you have the foundation that you need to begin your practice and delve further into the specific principles of T'ai Chi.

Chapter 4

Sowing Your T'ai Chi Seeds Mindfully

- -

In This Chapter

▶ Checking out the variables that make your practice more fruitful

▶ Minding your mind

▶ Battening down breathing

▶ Intensifying your practice — or not

- -

*I*n Chapter 3, you find out how to put down a strong foundation so you can build your T'ai Chi house with success. These concepts — from breathing to finding your energy — are key to any mind-body practice, let alone internal Chinese practices such as T'ai Chi.

In this chapter, I explain three elements that can help you fully realize the physical and mindful benefits of T'ai Chi. (These three actually apply to any mind-body practice.) Without building a foundation and applying these elements to your practice, T'ai Chi can become a simple physical dance. A dance is a beautiful thing to look at, but it lacks the depth and breadth that gives T'ai Chi its inner beauty — and allows you to experience the inner beauty that can enrich your daily life.

Sizing Up the Key Elements

When you consider the studies concerning mind-body practices, you may notice that many variables are tossed around as being central to finding mindfulness in any movement practice. (See Chapter 2 for more details on mind-body research.) But when you sift out the variables that are mostly twaddle or don't have a lot of reasoning behind them, you can see that the following elements stand true:

- Mindfulness
- Breath work
- Muscle use

If you apply these three elements to your T'ai Chi practice, you can gain health and fitness benefits for your body *and* your mind. These three are key and borne out by scientific research, but there are, of course, more you may discover as you deepen your practice.

Minding Yourself

I talk a lot about using your mind and your body. You can practice T'ai Chi — as well as Yoga or other mindful movement methods — in two ways:

- **Physically:** You basically crank out movements or forms to get a good workout, a nice stretch, or some pleasant exercise.
- **Physically *and* mindfully:** You use your body physically, but you also use your mind in a meditative and inwardly focused manner during all movements and forms.

To get the benefits that can reach far beyond the results of a nice workout, applying a meditative manner and an inward focus is the way to go.

Breathing through the Forms

Breathe, schmeathe . . . you may be getting a little tired of me talking about breathing! But I don't stop, because breathing fully and deeply makes or breaks the mind-body practice.

Keep in mind the following points:

- **You breathe only when you have to.** Those breaths are prompted by your body's involuntary need to suck in oxygen to survive and no conscious effort on your part as a part of movements or otherwise.
- **You exhale and inhale fully as you do the movements.** When moving through the forms, breathing is as important as the movements. Instructors and books prompt you to breathe, especially in particular places, while moving through forms.

One other thing: Tai Chi's breathing comes from the Dan Tien (an area close to what other movement forms may call your "core" or belly). For more on the Dan Tien, see Chapter 13. All movement comes from breath that comes from your Dan Tien.

Muscling Up to the Movements

Meditation is mindful and can be a vital part of any practice. But if you just *sit* and meditate — which is certainly a beneficial practice — you miss a certain component — movement. Add some movement, which uses muscle and adds some intensity at even low levels, and you may realize other benefits. You can do some minor movements, which don't have to include high-intensity push-ups and maniacally jumping around. Just lightly use your muscles in some way.

Balancing your fitness checkbook

I'm not suggesting that meditation is bad and that you shouldn't do it. Absolutely not! Meditation may be a great adjunct to many mind-body practices. But studies suggest that a small amount of movement can get you where you may want to go more quickly — depending, of course, on where you want to go.

Some Qigong movements — even a couple that I present in Chapter 14 — use such minor amounts of muscle that they are best used as a part of an entire practice.

You don't have to move about dynamically everyday. An entire practice is what you do as a lifestyle. Think of your practice as a checkbook that has to be balanced. One day you may only meditate, the next day you may move lightly, and the next day you may move more quickly. At the end of the week or month, if the combination of movement is balanced, you come out on top!

Intensifying or not

Then there's the question of aerobic intensity. In Chapter 2, I explain the traditional and non-traditional ways to look at aerobic exercise, as well as how that applies to T'ai Chi and other mind-body practices. If you do any traditional exercise, such as walking or aerobics, you are familiar with the health and weight-loss benefits. And traditional exercises can be nice supplements to mind-body practices like T'ai Chi because you can gain more benefits, such as combating osteoporosis or losing weight.

Picking up the intensity a notch

I admit that I'm an aerobic animal. I like feeling my heart beat go faster and challenging myself to work a little harder. I like the feeling of sweat dripping off my forehead. But I've also discovered the pleasures of a balanced regimen.

When you need to go slow, go really slow and enjoy it. When you want to go hard, go really hard and enjoy that, too. If you've picked up this book, you're likely ready for the *yin* and *yang* (the concept of opposites; see Chapter 3) in your fitness life. Or you at least you want to know more

about this concept to offset any skepticism about what it can do for you. Perhaps you doubt whether you can get enough out of going slower or less intensely. Take my word for it: You can. You may be surprised how much it can do for you. For more on that, take a look at Chapter 2. And if you're an aerobic animal, too, you may find that less — and a better balance — can mean more to your training. You may also find that discovering the mindful element and adding it to the physical element takes you farther more quickly.

T'ai Chi may not be high-intensity, and that's okay. You can do Tai Chi at a very low level (which is perfect for seniors or someone new to exercise) or at a pretty high level (which is great for adding mindfulness to an athlete's training or for balancing the lifestyle of someone who does traditional exercise).

The intensity you achieve during forms depends on the following factors:

- What style or school you choose
- How often you do the forms
- How many times you repeat the forms at one time
- How low you bend your knees or sink

Research suggests that a low to low-moderate intensity is best. Dump the heart rate calculations for a moment and just think about how you feel. If you rate how you feel on a scale of 0 to 10 (with 0 being so easy it's as if you're lying in bed and 10 being so hard that you may fall over exhausted), your feeling of effort during movement shouldn't exceed about 5.

Remember, though, that T'ai Chi isn't really about heart rates and such stuff, but rather about feeling and focus. Don't forget that fact as you move forward along the Eastern path.

Part II
Preparing to T'ai One On

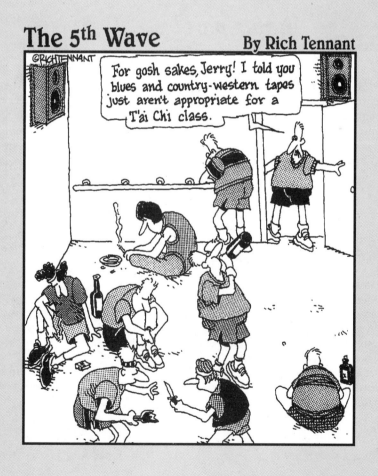

The 5th Wave   By Rich Tennant

©RICHTENNANT

For gosh sakes, Jerry! I told you blues and country-western tapes just aren't appropriate for a T'ai Chi class.

In this part . . .

1 show you the basic principles and background of T'ai Chi. Even if you aren't a big history buff, knowing a little bit about the history can help you understand the moves, because T'ai Chi is based on a lot of ancient history that can shed some fascinating light on the forms. In this part, you gain a better knowledge of the different parts of a full T'ai Chi practice as well as some insights into the basic principles of moving through T'ai Chi. If you read only one thing in this part, flip to the principles in Chapter 7. You need to grasp these principles to successfully do the movements.

Chapter 5

Saying Hello to the Founding Families

In This Chapter

▶ Meeting the historical families of T'ai Chi

▶ Deciding to do the Chen, Yang, Wu, or others

▶ Looking at the differences between the schools of T'ai Chi

*W*ith this book in hand, you're likely not looking for hundreds of pages of deep historical significance, tales of the Chinese fathers who developed T'ai Chi, and detailed charts showing the family trees of T'ai Chi ancestors.

Nevertheless, knowing a little bit about the background of the T'ai Chi practice can give you some perspective on the movements themselves and why it's done as it is today. I suppose that T'ai Chi is kind of like gourmet dining. (I don't know why I always use these food analogies.) If you see Boeuf Bourguignon on a menu but you don't speak or understand French, you may be a bit puzzled. But if you find out that it means "beef burgundy" and the recipe contains some red wine (burgundy!), you can then better understand what it may be like to order.

You don't have to know the entire ingredient list of Boeuf Bourguignon to be a gourmet diner, do you? Nope, just the basics. The same goes for T'ai Chi, especially as a novice. If you know just a little about the roots of T'ai Chi, you can approach your practice with a little more appreciation for its tradition and its beauty.

Fancying the T'ai Chi Tales

T'ai Chi's origins abound in tales and myths: Some are quite fanciful (and a heck of a lot of fun to read) but not necessarily substantiated.

If you choose to read more about T'ai Chi as your practice develops, enjoy the tales. Appreciate them for their stories but not necessarily for their truth.

Staying alive . . . and awake

The origin of Chinese martial arts training, which I explain in Chapter 1, is generally attributed to Bodhidharma ("Da Mo," in Chinese). He was a Buddhist monk who came to China from India in the sixth century A.D. Da Mo then arrived at the Shaolin monastery in Henan province in northern China.

Displeased by the physical weakness that often led his monks to nod off during study and meditation, Da Mo devised a series of temple exercises to strengthen and invigorate the monks. These exercises later became the movements of the Shaolin system, the Kung Fu (kung-*foo*) styles that imitate the fighting qualities of five animals: crane, snake, leopard, tiger, and dragon.

The moral here: Don't fall asleep in a class or in a meeting at work. You may find yourself being forced into exercise! No, no, just kidding.

Combating snakes and cranes

Chang San-Feng, a Taoist priest, was a student of the Shaolin temple in the thirteenth to fourteenth centuries, some seven-plus centuries after Da Mo kept his monks awake with kicking, twisting, and turning movements called by different names.

Legend holds that one day, Chang was awakened by the sounds of a snake and a crane (or a magpie, depending on which version you hear) engaged in mortal combat. (I'm not sure what that sounds like, but he must have recognized it.)

Fascinated, Chang watched as the snake moved smoothly and gracefully. It circled around, pulled back during an attempted strike, and then struck itself, never losing the beautiful circular smoothness. The crane (or was it a magpie?), on the other hand, was hard and linear. It snapped forward and struck right and left, nearly throwing itself off balance and being caught by surprise by the snake's smooth attacks.

Finally, the crane grew tired and tried to fly away. But the bird was already so tired because it didn't reserve any energy during the attacks for a retreating flight. All the snake had to do is strike only one well-placed and effortless blow, and it killed the bird, which was much larger than the snake.

Oh, there are other renditions to this story too, because legends are told and retold and change over the years with each retelling. For example, you may also hear that neither actually ever gained an advantage as they fought from dawn until dusk. The snake curled and coiled to avoid the sharp attacks of the bird's beak, while the bird used the softness of its flapping wings to fend off the snake's attempts. In the first version, the snake's softness won over the bird's hardness, while in this version, both used hard and soft to continue the battle.

Being a thoughtful monk, Chang realized that he had seen something that was more than merely snake and bird combat. He witnessed the soft, supple, energy-conserving, flowing, circular movements of the snake overcome the hard, linear, aggressive, energy-intensive attacks of the crane. He realized that men could likely use this type of system! I think that this was the big ah-ha moment. Of course, he could have also had the ah-ha moment when he saw the softness of both the snake and the bird used to an advantage in the second version, but does it really matter which version he really saw? Either way, they are great stories — Chang saw the advantage of softness and his proverbial light bulb went on.

Chang wasted no time devising a system of self defense based on this type of battle. Being a good monk, he also realized how other Taoist principles related so much to this system. Thus, T'ai Chi was born into this world as a movement and martial art for humans.

Savoring More Styles and Schools

Ah! Snakes flowing and cranes (or magpies) jabbing and stabbing — that sounds spectacularly simple. So you tell yourself and say to your friends and family, "I want to practice T'ai Chi."

What do you say when someone responds to your eager statement with the simple question, "What kind?"

"Huh?" you may ask, rather stunned. "What do you mean, 'What kind?' The kind like when the snake won the battle against the bird, of course!"

Ah, little Grasshopper, that's like saying that you want to buy a car. But what kind? A truck? A convertible? An SUV? A compact? A beat-up old Volkswagen bug, maybe?

Despite all the choices, you may not have the ability to make a reasonable choice. If you've never driven an SUV or a VW bug, how can you make a sound decision? Or know enough to decide what style you like best?

The same thing may happen if you go searching for a T'ai Chi school or instructor. You may not know enough about the school or the instructor to make a reasonable decision. Or you may have to take what you can find — like having the choice between driving a truck or, well, a truck.

In this book, I present mostly one school of T'ai Chi. A dictatorial sort of thing, huh? Be aware that I haven't chosen Yang style randomly. Yang style is the most common style taught in the United States, and you may not have a real choice. Nonetheless, you want to be aware of the options so you're not confused when a fellow practitioner talks about the Yang form, or the short form, or the Chen school, or whatever.

T'ai Chi history can be told many different ways, and names get spelled differently, sometimes depending on who handed down the story. Heck, no one's really sure about all this stuff anyway, so the dates may even vary a bit. Take in the historical information as if you're looking at a large map for an overview of the world.

Regardless of the style, all T'ai Chi schools insist on utilizing the proper mind-body principles of T'ai Chi. (You can find these principles in Chapter 7.) Without the proper principles in place, your T'ai Chi practice becomes mere calisthenics that look cool.

Clambering for Chen

The Chen style is to T'ai Chi what Shakespeare is to contemporary theater. Most of T'ai Chi stems from the Chen style (in the same way that contemporary theater has a basis in Shakespeare). Although the Chen style may not be as commonly practiced as other forms these days, it remains in about the second or third rung of popularity.

Developer and military officer Chen Wangting lived around 1600, during the Ming Dynasty. He was a soldier and a farmer, as well as a martial arts practitioner. Based on his needs as a soldier, he developed a system that combined the soft and supple movements that Chang saw in the snake-bird battle, with some faster and harder strikes and leaps.

For decades, the forms that he created were handed down from generation to generation, staying solely in the Chen family. The section "Flowing with Yang," later in the chapter, explains what happens next.

Some parts of Chen style are more explosive than the styles of the "typical" T'ai Chi discipline. Chen begins in slow, flowing movements and bursts into broad, big, attacking movements. The stances are low to the ground.

Flowing with Yang

Yang Luchan came to the Henan village in the 1800s. He was from a poor family and became an apprentice to the family at the age of 10. At that time, family outsiders were still not permitted to learn T'ai Chi. But that didn't stop little Yang. He did what any eager young boy would do — he found a crack in the wall! From that vantage point, he watched the Chen family practice at night. After thinking about what he saw, he practiced on his own to perfect the moves, adding his own style.

One day, Chen ordered Yang to spar with all the Chen students. One by one, Yang defeated each of them. Now that must have been a bit embarrassing to the Chen family! As a result, Yang began to teach his powerful and flowing Yang style in earnest.

At the age of 40, Yang went back to his home in the Hebei province to earn his living as a T'ai Chi teacher. He soon became an exceptionally well-known and well-respected T'ai Chi practitioner and teacher, as did his son (Yang Jianhou) and his grandson (Yang Chengfu). They both continued the lineage and developing the style and its name. In fact, there are of course flavors of both the son and grandson in the popular T'ai Chi taught today that is originally and historically based on the Yang Luchan style, which was to develop movements that were less difficult and easier for the masses.

If you take T'ai Chi in the Western world, you are most likely to experience the *Yang 24-Movement Form* (as I describe in Chapters 9 through 11). This style is the modified version of the original form with 108 movements. But you can also find forms of other numbers and lengths that teachers and schools have modified over the years.

Yang style has an even tempo with larger and tighter circular movements than the Chen style. The forms incorporate very large movements known for their flow from one move to the other. They're also simpler than other forms. The stances are middle height, not too low or too high, and they can be adjusted based on need and ability.

Honing Wu/Hao

Every student has to make his mark. Wu Yuxiang was a student of Yang (the father) in the 1800s, and he worked hard to reach perfection as well as develop his own version. He not only studied with Yang but also studied another, slightly different Chen style with one of Chen's nephews.

Hence, another style was born and bred — Wu. But it's sometimes called Hao. Or it's sometimes even called Wu/Hao, as I do. That's because there are two Wu styles (see "Bursting into Wu," later in this chapter). The Chinese names so boggle Western minds and eyes that the two founders' names couldn't be distinguished so easily. Hao Weizhen is the man credited with popularizing this form. So the Wu of Wu Yuxiang became commonly known as Wu/Hao. Now Hao about that.

The Wu/Hao style — the fourth most popular of styles but the third oldest — is a very refined form of T'ai Chi. Its moves are the smallest — very subtle — and some describe it as being the closest of all styles to meditation.

Discovering others under the sun

Chen and Yang are the most common styles and Wu/Hao is the next oldest, but you may find similar styles that have been altered through years of study, teaching, stylizing, and personalizing.

As with Yoga, dance, or any other kind of movement art, your T'ai Chi teacher may have a touch of his or her own style that you may feather to — or not.

No style is truly wrong, as long as it adheres to solid basics of correct postures and principles. It may just be a different road, all of which lead to the ultimate goal of higher awareness. You have to determine which style feels best to you and helps you get on that road.

Stylizing Sun

Sun style is a combination of the styles of many teachers. Sun originally was a master of fistfighting. In Beijing, he learned from Hao and developed his own style. Look for quickly moving hands combined with slow and gentle leg movements.

Bursting into Wu

You may see another style called Wu. For example, Wu Jianquan came a few decades later than the Wu/Hao style.

This Wu style has taller stances and smaller circular forms than the Chen and Yang styles. When practicing Wu, you lean forward slightly, as if reaching from the waist, and the movements follow each other rapidly. This style is probably the third most popular style today. There are some practitioners who hold that this Wu style is really just a variation on the popular Yang style.

Chapter 6

Scaling the Peaks of T'ai Chi Practice

- -

In This Chapter

▶ Forming your T'ai Chi forms patiently and practically

▶ Understanding the names

▶ Exploring other ways to move

▶ Practicing with a partner

▶ Considering if you want to wield weapons someday

- -

*T*his book is mostly about T'ai Chi *forms* — the flowing sequences of moving meditation — and I'm sure you're eager to get on with it. I start here introducing the T'ai Chi principles and forms that you read about in Chapters 7 through 11. But a T'ai Chi practice also has other parts — peaks, if you will — which you can either walk around or scale, depending on your time, interest, and dedication.

In this chapter, I first discuss the basics of T'ai Chi — that's the first peak in the mountain range. It's also the reason you're here, isn't it? I also briefly introduce three other peaks that you can climb to maximize your practice (that is, to complete your climb to the summit).

The other three areas are Qigong, Push Hands, and weapons practice. There is also another area — a much deeper study of T'ai Chi's classical philosophy. Because that study can demand a lifetime of work, I offer only a short section on it. If you find the Taoist quotes or other bits of philosophy in this book appealing to you, the classics may be an area you choose to explore further.

Taking Shape with T'ai Chi Forms

What most people commonly think of if they know a little something about T'ai Chi are the movements (see Chapters 8 through 11). But T'ai Chi isn't just about moving in interesting ways with your body (making the shapes of

T'ai Chi). You actually build on the principles of mindful movement (see Chapter 7) so you can gain benefits. (See Chapters 2 and 4 for more details on benefits.)

No matter how far along you are or will become in T'ai Chi practice, remember one thing: Every movement in T'ai Chi has its origin in some martial application. (If you want a reminder, turn to Chapter 5 and read about the snake and the crane in mortal combat.) Sure, the movements look pretty. They flow. They look graceful. But behind the curtain of beauty, the movements are self-defense applications. Knowing this information can help you learn the movements even if you never plan to do combat with them, because you know *why* you pull back or *why* you place a hand in front of your face.

Focusing on forms

Learning a single move in isolation is one thing. But learning an entire series of forms (or movements) that make up an entire sequence is an entirely different thing. Imagine learning the waltz. You pick up one box step just dandy. But what happens when you want not only to string together a whole bunch of steps but also to flow while you're doing them? To find the flow in T'ai Chi — as in waltzing — and the energy needed to achieve it, you need to learn entire sequences, not just one itty-bitty step in isolation.

Now, I don't mean that you need to learn all the steps at once! T'ai Chi is a lifetime practice. But if you aren't ready to dedicate your life, you can practice a few minutes every few days or an hour or two a week so you can learn the techniques of the forms and their sequencing.

Practicing patiently

Practice is a vital part of learning not only the physical part of T'ai Chi (see Chapters 8 through 11) but also the internal part of T'ai Chi. You can find out about T'ai Chi principles in Chapter 7, and you can refer to Chapters 3 and 4 for building a mind-body foundation.

At first, you may only be able to do one or two movements. But practice and patience brings you closer to the true feel. After you get there, you may be surprised how short one form, or *sequence,* is. Without pausing, it may only take 4 or 5 minutes. But if you go slowly (see Chapter 7 for the importance of going slowly), you may take up to a half-hour to do the form.

The forms are your alphabet, and after they become linked, they are your T'ai Chi vocabulary. All together, the forms are indispensable for developing balance, honing coordination, and building strength. (See Chapter 2 for health and science information.) They also help you move the chi within your body. (You can find more information about chi in Chapter 3.) Forms help you fine-tune the energy flow that helps unblock chi in your body.

Practicing principles

Forms also provide an excellent vehicle for learning to apply the principles of T'ai Chi. Although you may come to T'ai Chi for the movement, you may find that you want stay for the principles and the internal changes that you experience. Nothing gives you a better chance to work on the principles than the forms.

Knowledge of the forms is essential to learning to move with the physical and mental relaxation that T'ai Chi requires. Forms practice requires and develops the ability to "tighten the mind," as my collaborator Manny likes to say, which is the ability to maintain concentration on the task at hand. Simply put, you can't practice good T'ai Chi — physically or mindfully — while making a mental shopping list or worrying about your next project at work.

Practicing for proficiency

T'ai Chi practice requires focus because you have to develop proficiency doing the basic forms before you can really take on other things like sparring sequences, Push Hands, or weapons — a couple of the other T'ai Chi peaks that you may choose to one day summit. Simple Qigong is a different matter (I discuss Qigong in the following section, "Discovering the Charge of Qigong."), but more advanced Qigong may take more time and proficiency also.

Heck, doing the forms is like taking an art class. Instead of sketching stick figures and drawing sheet after sheet of trees, you want to do full landscapes dotted with picnicking people! However, if you can't draw a good tree or manage more than stick figures, your landscape won't be much to look at.

The same thing happens in T'ai Chi: If you don't apply the principles well, if you can't do the basic transitions or stances, you can't truly manage an entire sequence. Deficiencies in technique surface during the practice of flowing forms.

Training in forms lays a sound physical and mental foundation for everything you do in T'ai Chi. It allows you to work on the opening of the joints, the stretching of the muscles, and the development of *song* (pronounced *sung*). Song refers to relaxing and sinking your body lower. (See Chapter 7 for more details on the sinking feeling.) Maintaining mental focus ensures that the mind and body work together harmoniously.

Sifting through seemingly strange names

The names of the movements vary among styles or even among teachers of the same style. In Chapters 8 through 11, where I introduce the physical movement of forms, I give you some variations that you may hear.

But with or without variations, the names may sound rather odd, exotic, or even random to Western ears, and they may sometimes produce an inner smirk. (Repulsing a monkey? What does *that* mean? You can find out in Chapter 9.) But the names served an important purpose in the early days of T'ai Chi. For example, instead of describing all the components of a particular technique during a form, the teacher just said, "White Crane Cools Its Wings," and the students knew to assume a particular posture. Notice that the names generally describe the movement's quality, structure, and appearance. I also try to point out some connection between the name and where in the form you see the namesake appear occasionally.

Nevertheless, don't get all tied up in knots about the accuracy of the name. It is what it is. The particulars about the mindful and internal nature of T'ai Chi are far more important. A rose is a rose, you know?

Discovering the Charge of Qigong

Qigong (chee-*gung*) covers a lot of different types of movements and practices that involve using and feeling the body's energy. That can include being healed by someone else's energy (way beyond the scope of this book), passively meditating in a way that unblocks and uses your energy better (a bit closer to the intent here), and moving in a meditative way that unblocks your energy channels. That's more what this book is about!

The whole point of Qigong is to work with your *energy* — that's the *qi* (chee) part, which is just another spelling of chi (the word you more commonly see in the West) — to get it to move better so you can feel better and be healthier. You can find some information about chi and the channels through which chi flows in Chapter 3, as well as in the Qigong chapter, which is Chapter 13.

Qigong has innumerable systems — health, medical, spiritual, and even combat-oriented systems — that advocate perhaps hundreds or even thousands of movements and even some passive and non-moving practices. And different teachers and different schools all find what they think are the best ways to accomplish the goal of tapping into the energy.

All of this information can be pretty bewildering to the beginning student! Where do you start? What, if anything, do you add to a T'ai Chi practice? Why should I add something? In Chapters 13 and 14, you can find a lengthier introduction to Qigong, as well as some movements that you can try alone or as a part of your T'ai Chi practice.

For now, realize the following about Qigong:

> ✔ Qigong is an important element of a full T'ai Chi practice.
>
> ✔ You can choose to do more, less, or none of the movements depending on your needs, time, and focus.
>
> ✔ You may find that Qigong can help you perform better T'ai Chi.

Some people believe that T'ai Chi itself is a complex form of Qigong. Other purists disagree, believing they are separate and distinct mindful arts. But just as modern dance is an offshoot of ballet, both parts can be important if you want to fully delve into, explore, and learn the art.

With so many styles and movements to choose from, there is most certainly a Qigong style for everyone. All it takes is a willingness to explore.

Sparring Without Brute Force: Push Hands

You may decide that a few T'ai Chi forms are the extent of your practice. These forms may be the highest level that you want to go. They may give you what you feel you need. And you may be content with that achievement. T'ai Chi forms practice can provide enough challenge for a lifetime of study. And you can derive all the health benefits of T'ai Chi practice from the forms.

Ah, but you can choose to take another step. If you want to take the step that can help you fully realize all the lessons that T'ai Chi has to offer, you may want to move on to Push Hands.

Doubling up for double the benefits

Push Hands is a form of controlled and slow-moving T'ai Chi sparring in which you try to upset your opponent's balance while striving to maintain your own. Push Hands isn't as well-known as regular solo T'ai Chi, probably because it is a more advanced skill and requires two people. Finding a partner can be the tough part. The partner needs to be of similar ability, serving as an equal "sparring" partner. Or he or she can be of superior ability, serving as a teacher. On the other hand, once you become good enough, you can be a partner for someone of lesser ability, using the demand to be a teacher as a way to fine-tune your own ability. After you find a partner, you can try the drill in the section "Trying a little Push Hands" in this chapter.

But before you take on a duet form, you must first understand and internally practice the basic concepts on your own. That's because a duet drill requires you to go beyond "listening" to yourself and your energy, and to actually in some ways "listen" or feel your partner's energy. That comes in part through your hands, and promotes incredible sensitivity to another, as well as even more sensitivity to yourself.

In a much lesser way, Push Hands is like running your open palm over a heater. You can sense the energy of the warmth in your palm getting stronger as you're closer to the heat source, and then getting weaker as your hand gets farther away.

You may think that you have all the skills of T'ai Chi down pat — such as relaxation, body placement, balance, and energy flow — but until you're tested by a partner at your side, you can never realize how tense or unbalanced that you may actually still be! That is why the duet of Push Hands can help deepen your understanding of your T'ai Chi skills. You gotta get it right or you fall over. And the harder you try externally not to fall over, the more you tense up and, well, fall over.

Manny, my collaborator, points to a maxim in T'ai Chi for comparison: "Learning the form guides you to knowledge of yourself. Push Hands teaches you to know others."

Push Hands training is the acid test of relaxation. When performing the solo form, you can easily convince yourself that you are truly relaxed. But when you are faced with an opponent who is attempting to push you over, you soon discover whether you are indeed relaxed. Muscular tension manifested anywhere in the body gives a seasoned opponent a foothold and upsets your body's structure. When you can remain completely relaxed in the face of those efforts that should upset you, you can't be unearthed and upended. Your opponent appears to be trying to push a cloud or catch a feather wafting through the air.

Manny tells the story of performing Push Hands with his teacher: No matter how hard Manny tried, his teacher sent him flying. But when Manny stopped trying so hard, he actually succeeded in knocking over his teacher. That's because he stopped thinking about the *goal* — to get even and send his teacher flying — and, instead, concentrated on his balance and internal power.

Sensitizing your sensitivity with four skills

The goal of Push Hands is to develop sensitivity of your opponent and the attack, to yield to it, and then to respond to it appropriately when the opening to do so presents itself. In other words, wait for the weak spot and then jump in with both feet — or hands.

Table 6-1 explains the four energies that you need when facing your partner-opponent. *Partner*-opponent? It was simply *opponent* a moment ago! Any adversary is really just a partner whom you can use to practice your skills. Thinking this way can actually set you free from aggressive feelings that can cloud your perception.

Table 6-1		Four Energies
Energy	*Translation*	*Ability*
Ting Jing	Listening energy	The ability to hear with your ears and, more importantly, to have the sensitivity in the hands and eventually in the entire body to "hear" and receive the opponent's touch with full awareness. This is only possible when the mind and body are profoundly relaxed and aware.
Dong Jing	Understanding energy	The ability to sense your partner's intention as soon as he or she touches you. Push Hands allows you to sense where your partner intends to direct his or her energy against you. Again, you can only achieve this if you are truly relaxed.
Hua Jing	Neutralizing energy	The ability to divert the force of your partner's push through the application of timing, angles, and circular movement. This skill allows you to yield to your partner's attack while maintaining contact. In Push Hands, you should not feel pressure build up at the point of bodily contact or lose contact entirely. By maintaining relaxed contact (see Dong Jing), you can sense when it is time to apply the fourth skill
Fa Jing	Discharging energy	The ability to apply your force to the partner-opponent when you are put in a disadvantage and can't receive it well. When you are able to yield properly, you are able to lead your partner into an off-balance position. At this point, a slight application of force is enough to break the opponent's root. Then you can send your opponent flying, so to speak!

Here's how you apply the four energies:

1. **Your "listening energy" allows you to receive your opponent's touch with full awareness.**

2. **Your "understanding energy" lets you sense what the opponent intends to do.**

3. **Use "neutralizing energy" to maintain contact while you absorb and redirect the opponent's force without giving him or her a solid place to push against.**

4. **Lead the opponent into a disadvantaged position and apply "discharging energy" to push him or her away with relatively little effort.**

As Manny's teacher used to say, "When someone comes at you, let him come in. Then just get out of his way and help him get where he's going more quickly."

Trying a little Push Hands

Talk a friend or T'ai Chi colleague into trying this movement with you. Keep in mind that a true Push Hands routine can be complicated because it involves some of the basic forms. You can be better if you already have some familiarity with the skills in this chapter, as well as the basic principles of T'ai Chi. But for now, try the following movement:

1. **Stand facing your partner, both of you in a Bow Stance with the left foot forward. (Your left foot is in front of your partner's right hip and vice-versa.) Stand with your left arms forward in a Ward-Off position (see Chapter 9) with the back of your hands in contact (see Figure 6-1).**

2. **While keeping your hands in constant contact, one of you shifts your weight slightly backward onto the right foot while turning your body to the right at the waist.**

3. **When you are as far back as you can go while maintaining good form, turn to the left at the waist and shift your weight forward to the left foot. Your partner moves with you, going forward (advancing) when you go backward (retreating) and vice-versa as you alternate the push-and-pull. Keep the hands touching without being knocked off balance.**

   If the contact breaks, your sensitivity to the energy was not good. If pressure builds at the point of contact, it means that your retreating partner isn't yielding enough.

4. **Continue this for several minutes and then repeat this movement with your right foot forward in a Bow Stance and the right arms forward.**

If you want to find out more about Push Hands movements, refer to some texts in the Appendix.

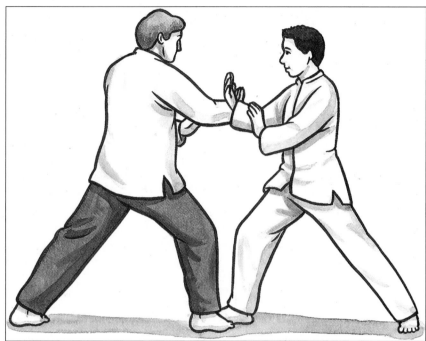

Figure 6-1:
Partnering
up with
Push Hands.

Wielding Weapons

Now, wait a minute, what do weapons have to do with mindful and peaceful T'ai Chi? That may be what you're asking yourself, huh? Because you most likely don't intend to do battle, perhaps you should skip this part of T'ai Chi practice.

Early T'ai Chi practitioners sometimes found themselves needing to defend themselves using swords and spears, but that simply isn't the case in this day and age. Firearms have long since replaced swords and spears as the most common weapons.

Nonetheless, weapons training can be a relevant part of T'ai Chi practice. You don't find any weapons instruction in this book, because it is an advanced level of practice. But in this section, I describe the different weapons and provide you with reasons weapons training can bring the serious student to higher levels of proficiency, mindfulness, and health.

Plus, using a weapon can serve to actually extend your chi beyond the body to the end of the weapon.

Benefiting from weapons

You can experience two primary benefits with weapons training:

- ✔ Discipline
- ✔ Body awareness

First and foremost, training with weapons teaches discipline. Certainly, all T'ai Chi training requires discipline, but weapons training requires a special discipline. For one thing, you're kind of swinging a potentially dangerous tool around your body. That takes great care and concentration, particularly if you're performing a training exercise with a partner. You don't want to slice anybody up, do you?

Weapons training is a particularly fine platform for discovering how to "tighten your mind," which means focusing on the task at hand without letting yourself get distracted by little things fluttering around inside your brain as well as around you.

Weapons training also helps you develop greater awareness of your body and its movement. Extending a sword or spear outwards changes your center of gravity, so you're forced to pay attention to your body. And to stay upright, you have to make subtle adjustments to your placement and stance. This greater awareness carries over to your regular forms, as well as to any Push Hands training or Qigong that you may do.

Attaining more discipline and greater awareness together can translate into achieving higher levels of T'ai Chi ability.

Oh, and don't forget the basic principles of T'ai Chi (see Chapter 7), because weapons training needs to be performed with the same foundation. Otherwise, you may as well just swing a stick around you.

Typing the weapons

The following three weapons are most commonly used in T'ai Chi training:

- ✔ *Dao* (or broadsword)
- ✔ *Qiang* (or spear)
- ✔ *Jian* (or straightsword)

You may also find other weapons, such as the staff, used in other schools. But these three weapons are the most common. Each weapon requires a different technique and develops different skills. Generally, you learn them in order — Dao, spear, and then Jian. As the T'ai Chi saying goes, "While the Dao may be learned in one hundred days, the Jian takes ten thousand days."

Philosophizing over the classics

After you move through the forms, Push Hands, a little weaponry, and some other things, you may find that your curiosity is a smidgen piqued about the philosophy behind the forms. Listen to your curious intuition because it can expand your T'ai Chi horizons and help you understand even more about the forms, their practice, and their deeper meaning. You don't have to make an epic journey or learn Chinese to find out more about this philosophy. T'ai Chi and Taoist classics can light your way. Luckily, they are translated and mostly available in the West. Why read the classics and not just books that talk about them? For the same reason that you must read Shakespeare's plays (rather than texts about him) to get truly acquainted with the heart of the man.

The primary books for finding out about Taoism are the *Tao Te Ching*, the *I-Ching* (also called the *Book of Changes*), and the writings of Chuang-Tzu. You can find more information about these books in the Appendix. Because T'ai Chi is predicated upon Taoist philosophy, a good understanding of these books translates into a better understanding of T'ai Chi principles. To dig even deeper, you can seek out the classic treatises written by such early T'ai Chi masters as Chang San-Feng, Wong Chun-Yua, and Wu Yu-Hsiang (also sometimes written as Zhang Sanfeng, Wang Zongyue, and Wu Yuxiang). But you need to be dedicated! To the Western mind, these brief treatises can be obscure and hard to understand, although with patience and repeated reading, you can deepen your understanding of the deeper mysteries of T'ai Chi.

So why bother reading these perhaps obscure people and dusty texts? Because when you read the classics (they've been pretty popular in China for, oh, about 3,000 years), you get T'ai Chi philosophy in its purist state. When someone else attempts to translate the literature (that means me, too!), small things get twisted a little. One little twist here and there for a few centuries, and you can imagine what happens to the true meaning. To get to the marrow inside the bones, go to the old masters.

Doing the Dao

The *Dao* (pronounced *dow*), or broadsword, is a large, curved, single-edged weapon that is suited for cutting and slashing techniques (see Figure 6-2). It is wielded with circular, decisive techniques that require and build large amounts of circular energy. Practice with the Dao helps you become more aware of the energy generated by the weapon rather than the solo form. And being a heavier weapon, the Dao provides a sort of weight training that is oriented specifically to martial arts.

The strikes are delivered with the weight of the body behind each strike. Yet, the body must remain relaxed and rooted. Training with the Dao enables you to develop the ability to move quickly and deliver strikes with enormous force while remaining relaxed.

Figure 6-2:
My, that's a broad sword!

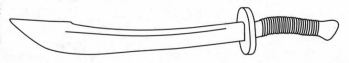

Savoring the spear

The Qiang (pronounced *kyang*), or spear, is a long weapon that is held with the right hand at the base of the spear with the left hand forward (see Figure 6-3). Training with the spear usually takes the form of solo exercises that are short combinations of techniques. These exercises generally consist of two blocking techniques and a thrust, and they are practiced over and over again for hundreds of repetitions, which helps develop the ability to discharge energy suddenly.

You can also do a two-person exercise in which you try to maintain contact with the opponent's spear. This exercise has some similarity to Push Hands training, but with a weapon. It further develops the ability to sense and respond to an opponent's intentions.

Figure 6-3:
Brandishing a spear . . . oh, dear!

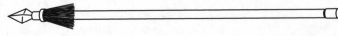

Jockeying with the Jian

The *Jian,* or straightsword, was traditionally regarded as the gentleman's weapon (see Figure 6-4). The Jian requires great care and subtle handling. No wonder. This sucker is sharpened on both sides of the blade! The movements of the Jian are not as sweeping or as heavy as the Dao's movements. The Jian relies more on the flexible movement of the wrist to perform the twisting, turning movements required to wield it effectively. Working with it can help develop quick and efficient footwork.

Figure 6-4:
Settling a score with a straight-sword? Don't even think about it!

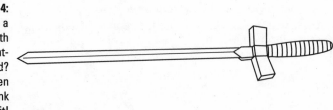

Chapter 7

Internalizing the Principles

- -

- -

T'ai Chi is not only about the *movements* (or forms), but about the *principles* by which you practice the movements. (See Chapters 9 through 11 for more details on the forms.) If you tap into the principles properly, you discover the stillness in the movement and, in turn, the energy that flows through your spirit. If you don't tap into the principles, T'ai Chi becomes nothing but a series of dance steps without a soul.

In this chapter, I give you the lowdown on T'ai Chi principles. These principles are not about looking pretty while you do the dance — although that's a nice side benefit. Instead, they help you focus on the internal aspects, which can provide you with health benefits (see Chapter 2 for more information on the benefits of T'ai Chi). You have to recognize the internal before you can begin to venture into the realms of energy and spirit.

Take heed of the ten T'ai Chi principles that I give you in this chapter. They go along with all the other information in this book about culture and history (see Chapter 5), as well as the basics and forms in Chapters 8 through 11.

Like the forms and names in T'ai Chi, the list of principles varies slightly depending on the school, teacher, or style. No set list is handed down from generation to generation — that would be way too convenient. But if you look and listen closely, you find that the core of any set of T'ai Chi principles is identical.

So don't just read these words. Think about and internalize them.

Slowing Down — Principle #1

If you get nothing else about T'ai Chi, get this: Go slowly. This, my little Grasshopper, is the Grand Ultimate Principle (if there was such a title). As you do T'ai Chi movements, pretend that you're the tortoise in the race against the hare. Rushing gets you nowhere — certainly not to a mindful balance and definitely not to enlightenment. I doubt that the Yogis on the mountains rushed to the top and missed the view along the way.

Think about what your body is doing and concentrate on what comes next. Slowing down also lets you have moments along the way to take stock of what your body is doing and feeling instead of zooming past that chance. In other words, slow down to smell the daisies.

On the first day of a Tae Kwon Do class that Manny took many years ago, the teacher started out explaining how the students would learn many stances in the first phase. One young woman then asked, "When will we start to learn jumping kicks?" The teacher responded, "You can't even walk properly yet, and you want to fly?"

Take the time to learn how to walk so you can indeed fly.

In contrast to the physical reasons for slowing down, going slower also leaves you time to experience a mindful calm, which may help you get your chi flowing correctly. That's the Grand Ultimate.

The stillness that comes with slowness is what is inherent in the movement of T'ai Chi. Find the stillness in your slow movement and the movement in the quiet stillness.

When Manny's classes practice a form, he tells the students, "First one done is a rotten egg." Ah, humor is a wonderful thing. No rotten eggs, okay?

Taking It Easy — Principle #2

In the Western world, forcing things is a way of life. Many people make things happen while tensing up or clenching — physically and/or mentally. The T'ai Chi mantra is the opposite of being tense: Take it easy. Be calm. Relax.

Look down at your hands. Perhaps your fingers are holding on to a pencil for dear life. What about your legs? Are they crossed tightly? Think about your shoulders. Up to your ears perhaps? Stop tensing. But that doesn't mean slouch on the couch. Although you want to avoid being as stiff as a plank, you don't want to be as limp as a cooked spaghetti noodle. Imagine being a snake — soft, supple, and relaxed but powerful to boot.

Perfectionists make poor T'ai Chi students

Do you want to know where every eyelash should fall when you do T'ai Chi? I can relate. I'm always asking, "Where?" But Manny points out that because perfectionists spend too much time worrying about getting the external movements right, they often lose focus on the bigger picture of the internal keys. Perfectionists can take longer to really get it; or they never get it (and then give up); or they eventually take the big step and let go of the perfectionism. Letting go can help in daily life, too.

Avoid focusing on the *external forms,* the body positioning and how it all looks. Instead, focus on the *internal forms,* the calm, relaxed, easy, deep-breathing movements based on the T'ai Chi principles. You need to perform the physical movements well, but if you get the internal stuff, you'll eventually get the movements. Manny says, "All of a sudden, it just falls into place."

Use your mind to relax the body, and use your body to relax the mind. You can't use brute force to learn the forms. If you relax and use only the exact amount of energy you need, you can probably learn the forms quicker — and better.

Holding extra tension in your body means expending extra energy, which you want to avoid in T'ai Chi. Save your energy for when you really need it — during your forms.

Thinking in Curves — Principle #3

Movement in T'ai Chi is curved and circular, rarely straight and linear. This allows one movement to flow seamlessly into the next.

Take a look at the famous yin-yang symbol in Figure 7-1. Nope, not a straight line in the place. The line separating white from black is curved, which represents cycles of change. Straight lines, on the other hand, indicate stagnation — sort of like a muck-covered pond in the park, which isn't what you want your insides to resemble.

From a martial arts perspective, the purpose of T'ai Chi's circular motion is to disguise from an opponent where a move stops and starts. That makes it easier to throw an opponent off and win a fight. Curved motion allows you to intercept the motions of your opponent and move with him or her. The curved blocks of T'ai Chi allow you to maintain contact with the opponent so you can better prevent the possibility of being caught unaware by another strike.

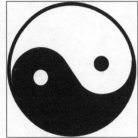

Figure 7-1:
The curved,
non-
stagnated
lines of yin
and yang.

From a mindful perspective, a rounded or curved joint or limb promotes better energy flow throughout your body. A sharply angled joint is like a soda straw bent over too far: Lemonade can't get up and into your mouth, no matter how hard you try.

In T'ai Chi practice, elbows aren't locked, not even during a push or punch. Knees aren't straightened, not even in a kick. Wrists aren't cocked forward or backward. At all times, avoid snapping out your joints. Keep them soft and curved.

When the chi flows smoothly, you'll realize why you worked on being curvy. And your insides will thank you for it.

Being Simple — Principle #4

Simplicity boils down to the ability to live fully and naturally, moving and feeling the way that feels best. This ability can be difficult for most people to attain, considering today's frenzied pace that encourages you to have one eye on tomorrow and your other eye on the cell phone.

T'ai Chi practice requires simplicity, but it also provides simplicity. It gives you an opportunity to put the world on hold for a while and let your mind settle into a simpler state.

Simplicity also refers to the ability to do things with as little effort as is necessary. You've likely seen pictures of amazing feats of strength displayed by people who don't look as if they could muster the strength to smoosh a spider. That's because these people dissect the task simply and use only the effort needed for the task at hand. They grab at a certain moment, in a specific way, and just push.

Simplicity also means to go with what feels natural to your body. If going from one form to another feels twisted or unnatural, it probably is. You're probably overthinking the move. Don't think. Shake out your mind. Then try again, letting your body move into the posture naturally — usually, you're doing it right! But don't try all night.

Avoid overanalyzing T'ai Chi. Keep it simple.

Sinking Lower — Principle #5

Bending your knees to sink lower — one of the keys of good T'ai Chi technique — isn't just about giving your legs a workout. As with other mind-body techniques, T'ai Chi is a process, not a goal for some kind of fitness. Fitness and strength happens. The demand to sink lower stems from T'ai Chi's roots in training for martial combat (see Chapter 5). If you can sink lower than your opponent, you can get beneath his or her center of gravity and turn him or her topsy-turvy. The higher a person stands, the easier he or she is to uproot.

Have you ever been on a boat while it rocked through the waves? Or on a bus or train that swayed along, perhaps jerking a bit in stops and starts? What do you naturally do to stay upright? You bend your knees. The same basic concept applies in T'ai Chi. Sinking lower allows you to root firmly to the floor or ground beneath you. You can also store a little energy in your coiled muscles and unleash it if you suddenly straighten or move. For example, if you try to jump up to make a 2-point basket, you bend your knees to go higher. But if you try to jump up from a straight-legged stance, you don't get very far.

Don't be afraid to push yourself a little. Try that sinking move. How about a little lower? Bend your knees naturally, but make sure that you don't let your butt stick out behind out or tuck it hard underneath you. The tailbone just relaxes downward for power and to avoid ending up in a swayback position.

When you first do T'ai Chi, your knees may be nearly straight because you lack of strength and flexibility. That's okay. As you progress, you will be able to bend your knees more. An advanced T'ai Chi practitioner is often quite low to the ground!

Don't bend your knees to the point of being uncomfortable. T'ai Chi is not about pain. Find a level that isn't too hard but still challenges you.

Sinking lower is also a behavioral characteristic honed in T'ai Chi. In other words, you retain an appropriately humble view of your own abilities, no matter how good you are. I'm sure that you've met people like that. You chat. The person seems nice enough. Then you find out later that she's won a Nobel Prize or written a bestseller or competed in the Olympics.

The philosophy of *Tao Te Ching* sagely says the following: "All rivers run to the sea because it is lower than they are. The ocean's willingness to be humbler and lower than the rivers gives it its power." (See the Appendix for more details on this source.)

Appreciating Opposites — Principle #6

All T'ai Chi forms and sequences are a combination of opposites, in the same way that all things in the universe are a cyclical interplay of opposites. Remembering the principle of opposites is a good way to keep track of where you are in a form — not to mention in life — and perhaps where you should go next. The forms always apply the principle of opposites — forward and back, weight-bearing or non-weight-bearing, force and stillness, high and low, reach and pull back, or lift and lower. You never go forward and then go forward again. A forward move is always followed by some kind of backward move that sort of winds up for the next forward move.

Think about playing baseball. After you swing the bat and hit the ball, you don't keep the bat in the forward position if you want to hit the ball again! You bring it back so you can bring it forward again.

These opposites underscore the ancient Chinese philosophy of yin and yang. Refer to Figure 7-1 for a look at the yin-yang symbol. *Yin* movements typically are receptive, non-weight-bearing, pulled back, and use or have more emotional energy. *Yang* movements are expansive, weight-bearing, attacking or reaching out, and use or have a more muscular energy. In Chinese philosophy, yin represents the feminine nature of the universe, and yang represents the masculine.

T'ai Chi tries to keep you balanced between the yin and yang of movement, creating a flowing, harmonious, and rhythmical dance — the dance of opposites. This harmony also applies to your life. If you create and maintain a fine harmony between the opposites in your character (for example, being orderly and allowing a little mess too, being fun-loving while enjoying seriousness), you become a healthier and more balanced person.

In *The Complete Book of T'ai Chi Chuan*, Wong Kiew Kit wrote, "If there is only yin and no yang, or vice versa, then that is not T'ai Chi Chuan." (See the Appendix for more information on this book.)

Staying Balanced — Principle #7

In T'ai Chi and in life, balance applies to everyone both physically and mentally. Physical balance is essential for proper performance of T'ai Chi. Heck, it's essential for walking down the hallway without falling over, or for hitting a tennis ball without landing on your face. T'ai Chi requires and provides not only simplicity (see "Being Simple — Principle #5," earlier in this chapter), but it also requires and provides balance. Studies show that seniors — or anybody needing better balance — can benefit from a T'ai Chi practice (see Chapter 2 for more details on research), but teachers themselves also see the positive differences in their students.

Manny has had a large number of senior citizens who, after several weeks of T'ai Chi classes, told him that their balance in day-to-day tasks and overall confidence in movement had improved. Why? Because T'ai Chi provides increased leg, hip, and abdominal strength; an improved awareness of body positioning; and an ability to move comfortably forwards, backwards, and laterally.

Many people think that physical balance comes naturally. But like aerobic fitness or leg strength, physical balance also needs practice to stay tuned. I discovered that several years ago when, as a nationally competitive athlete, I sprained my ankle and then kept turning it. I not only had to start doing balance drills, but I still do them today.

T'ai Chi also teaches balance in daily life. You discover how to live more centered and calm, avoiding both ends of the temperament scale.

Another philosophy of *Tao Te Ching* says the following: "The most opportune times to topple a tree are either when it is a sapling and easily uprooted, or when it is old and ready to fall. In the center between these extremes, it is hard to topple."

Moving the Whole Package — Principle #8

You've heard the little ditty, "The shin bone is connected to the knee bone; the knee bone is connected to the thigh bone." Well, that tune applies to T'ai Chi, too. Your whole body is one package, and any movement by one body party causes an action or reaction in another part of the body. You don't move a hand and then stand there and check it out; you don't move a foot and then stop to check it out. The body moves together, like a snake rhythmically slithering along (except you are upright).

When you were a kid, remember twisting up a wet towel and snapping it at your little brother or sister? You snapped your arm and wrist, and then the movement rolled out along the towel, snaking all the way to the end where it finally released its energy. In T'ai Chi, something similar happens in your body in a slower sense. The movement starts at one place (your feet grounded into the floor, for example) and reverberates up your legs, through your body, and out into your arms and hands.

Think unity, continuity and coordination. Without a unified and continuous coordination of movement, the action becomes disorderly. And you certainly don't want disorderly T'ai Chi!

Another aspect of the movement is its dimensionality. T'ai Chi is three-dimensional because the movements of your "whole package" occur in all planes simultaneously, sometimes spiraling around each other. The spiraling action is one way to create force with little effort. But this concept is not something that you likely get first time out of the gate. In fact, you don't want to get wrapped up in the technical part because your movements may become disjointed in the process of forcing them. (See "Taking It Easy — Principle #2," earlier in this chapter.)

Principally postural

In Chapter 8 you can find detailed instruction about the basic movements, including posture and stances. But posture also has basic principles that have to do with the mental aspects of T'ai Chi. The bottom line is that if you stand properly, you end up with better energy flow in your body because you connect to the earth better. And you don't have any "kinks" in your chi hose. Starting from the top of your body, the following list gives you key posture and body principles to follow during your practice:

✔ **Head is erect as if suspended by a string.** This allows the spirit to rise to the top of your body, or head, to help refresh you mentally.

✔ **Teeth touch lightly and are not clenched.** Clenched teeth block the chi flow.

✔ **Tongue touches the upper palate just behind the front teeth.** This connects two energy channels (see Chapter X) so the chi can circulate better between front and back.

✔ **Shoulders relax downward but aren't pulled forcefully downward.** Shoulders hiked up or forced downward can create muscular tension that can then move throughout your body, which in turn can cause chi to rise and weaken your body.

✔ **Body is held with "five bows."** This means a concave chest and elbows and knees softly bent. An extended chest causes chi to rush upward. As a result, you become top heavy, and it becomes harder to keep your feet rooted.

✔ **Tailbone tucked under and relaxed downward.** Again, no kinks in the hose. Combined with a tall head, this technique lengthens your spine and opens up your chi flow even more.

✔ **Knees bend but don't extend over your toes, and your weight sinks to the earth.** This principle makes sure that power is maintained with the flow.

✔ **Feet root firmly to the earth with body centered.** This principle allows you to connect the acupoint just behind the ball of the foot to the earth so you can soak up earth's chi into your body.

If you do all these principles properly, you are "solid as an oak tree" from the waist down and "light as a willow tree" from the waist up — you are maintaining the principle of opposites! (See "Appreciating Opposites — Principle #6," in this chapter.)

The late T'ai Chi Master Zhang Lu Ping knew the spiraling technique well. Manny had the "privilege of being thrown around by him" (his words, not mine!) at a weekend workshop. No matter how well Manny thought that he'd prepared a pending movement, he said that he was moved as easily as if he were a leaf, not a 175-pound man! By the time Zhang manifested the spiraling force up into his arms and hands, it contained an irresistible momentum.

When you discover how to move all the parts of your body in harmonious combination, your movements take on a surprising power.

Going with the Flow — Principle #9

T'ai Chi is about continuity and flow, without a break in time or space. Like balance (see the preceding principle), flow has both physical and mental qualities.

Physically, T'ai Chi movement is smooth, purring, and uninterrupted. Your legs, feet, and arms reach the final position at the same time, no matter how far they have to travel. But they don't ever just stop. In Chapters 8 through 11, I may call a place in a form an "end," but the forms don't really end. No dams along the T'ai Chi river exists to disrupt the flow. When you come to what seems like an end, you move through it and flow to the next place. But novices and Westerners unaccustomed to this style of movement are more comfortable thinking through a movement with a beginning and an ending before they can perceive it as one long flowing river.

Over time, the repetition of this type of flowing movement lets you manifest your chi.

Mentally, your mind must be placid and able to stay focused and aware of your body. The ability to go with the flow also carries over into your daily life. It can help you reduce day-to-day stress and strain. You figure out how to avoid struggling so hard, and you realize that riding the river's waves is a lot easier than swimming against them.

Here's a real-life lesson from Manny: "Growing up near the beach in South Carolina, we were always instructed that if we were caught in an undertow, we should swim with it until the current lessened so we could make it to the surface. The people who fought the undertow were the ones who drowned." So, he philosophizes, "Life is like that sometimes — events come along where you have no control. The only thing to do is ride with it until you can find your way out. That is much easier to do if you have a calm and relaxed mind that goes with the flow rather than a struggling mind that tries in vain to force something."

Staying Rooted — Principle #10

Even with your feet on the ground, you may sometimes find yourself off-balance or perhaps just fleetingly in one place. In T'ai Chi, you want to feel yourself firmly rooted to the ground with every step you take.

During T'ai Chi practice, your weight is centered between the ball of your foot and your heel, and squarely between each side. This centering is not only to make sure that your invisible but omnipresent opponent can't topple you with a little finger but also to make sure that the energy acupoint makes full contact with the earth and soaks in the chi that your body needs.

Try this drill that Manny's teacher used to have his class do. You need a partner to do this exercise. Start doing a series of forms. At some point, without warning, your partner calls out, "Stop." Wherever you are, you freeze the motion. You should be able to freeze without wobbling, falling over, or stuttering in any way. If you're able to do so, you are well-rooted and well-balanced. If not, you are using momentum, you aren't rooted so well, and you may be stepping out too far in forms.

Avoid sitting back on your heels or leaning forward on the balls of your feet. These positions are insecure, but not uncommon. You also want to avoid standing or walking with your weight rolled outward or inward on your feet. Heck, that can even hurt over time, whether you're walking through a park or doing T'ai Chi. And neither are supposed to hurt. Try just standing up then turning your senses to your feet. Where do you sense the pressure with the ground? Centered or on one side or another?

Master, how long will it take me to be the best?

A young man approached a respected karate master and asked him, "How long must I train to become the finest karate practitioner in all of Japan?"

"Ten years," said the master.

"Ten years is a long time," said the young man. "What if I practice twice as hard as anyone else?"

"Twenty years," said the master.

"What if I practice with all my might, day and night," the young man asked, "stopping only to eat and sleep?"

"Thirty years," said the master.

"Master," the young man exclaimed, "why is it that every time I say that I will work harder, you tell me it will take longer?"

"Because when one is fixed upon the goal," the master said, "there is only one eye left with which to find the way."

Part III
Knocking on T'ai Chi's Door

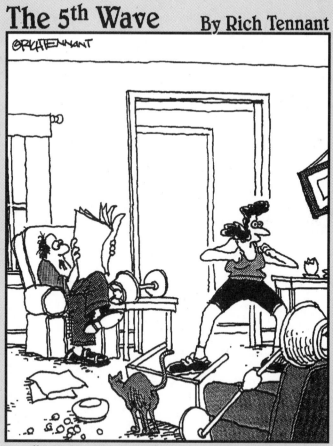

"I'm glad T'ai Chi relaxes YOU!"

In this part . . .

In the first two parts, you stepped up to T'ai Chi, shook its hand, and had a little chat about what it's all about. Perhaps you enjoyed learning about the traditions and some history, as well as about the principles that help you fully realize the mindful fruits of taking on T'ai Chi.

It's time to stand up and be counted.

This part is where you learn not only about the basic posture and breathing techniques, and other steps that are foundations to any T'ai Chi practice, but you also get to start moving through some sequences of forms, finding out how to link them so you truly can feel the flow. Look for the traditional Yang-style Short Form — which is long enough to break into three chapters — as well as a shorter form geared for novices, seniors, or anyone looking for a slightly easier way to get started.

Chapter 8

Building the Basics

T'ai Chi has a deep cultural background. And, before you know it, you can become immersed in the minute details of philosophy, language, culture, and history. All of that is indeed fascinating information — I introduce some of it in Parts I and II — and it can be a great way to find some perspective for the whats, whys, and hows of the movement itself.

But if you really want to practice T'ai Chi — and I do mean *do* the movement called T'ai Chi, not just read about it — you may as well stand up and get with it. There's nothing like first-hand experience to help spark even more interest in the cultural background for the whats, whys, and hows.

No matter what school you attend, teacher you study under, or style you learn, some concepts and steps will rise to the surface over and over. In this chapter I review those first, from how to stand and breathe to how to speak the T'ai Chi language of the position you're facing to how to hold your hands and feet.

Then, I show you how to apply some of these basics to a couple of transitional movements that surface again and again in many forms, including the ones that come up in Chapters 9 through 12.

After you have all that down, I tell you about a sequence — drill if you will — to help you learn the basics, and I show you how to warm up for your practice, too, based on real-life warm-ups that my collaborator Manny does regularly in the classes he teaches. This is where you get to move. So unglue yourself from the chair, find a nice open space that frees your mind, and take a deep breath. . . . You're ready to dive into T'ai Chi!

The basics in this chapter are all great stuff that will make your T'ai Chi practice and movement better, from the details about hands and feet, to instruction about transitions and warming up. But the first thing to remember is this: Don't get too wrapped up in the small stuff. If you spend all your time trying to figure out if your right toe is an inch too far to the left, you'll never get to experience the true feeling of T'ai Chi, and you'll certainly never learn to let your chi flow if your brain is too busy analyzing your body placement. So try to get the basics right, but let that flow too as your practice develops. All of it will come with time.

Tackling the Basics of the Basics

These two basics — posture and breathing — are actually basics to life, not just T'ai Chi. That is, by the way, one of the beauties of T'ai Chi — its concepts, principles, and basic constructs are things you can learn and apply almost immediately to your everyday life. So think of these two basics as helping you learn how to stand — and standing, as you well know, comes before learning to "walk so you can run." You also learn how to breath fully so you can also laugh at life better too.

T'ai Chi posture

Posture has probably been drilled into you since you were a small tyke, whether you actually paid attention or not. How many times have you heard someone tell you, "stand up tall," "sit straight," or "stop slouching?" Perhaps because of these corrections — or in spite of them — you developed one of the following possibilities:

- ✔ Great posture per the Western standard, which may mean a very tall and inflexible stance that requires you to "suck it in" all the time.

- ✔ Terrible posture that is now an ingrained part of your existence. Maybe you slouch through the back, drop your chest down, stick out your butt, or let your chin hang in front of your chest.

- ✔ An overly rigid military posture, which means you may stand tall, but your chest is puffed out and tense and your shoulders are pulled back tightly.

Unfortunately, none of these is a super posture for T'ai Chi, and the tension inherent in them may be the reason behind any kind of pain you may have in, for example, your back, shoulders, or neck.

Analyzing your normal posture

Before you can work into a great T'ai Chi Posture, take a moment to see if you can figure out what you're doing now.

Stand as you normally do. Now take a look at the curves through your spine — first while facing a mirror, then with your side to the mirror. The natural curves of your spine should remain — they enable your spine to be more forgiving of impact. (The curves that flow back and forth like a graceful S in the neck, middle back, and low back are important.) But ask yourself these questions as you scan down your body:

✔ Are the curves overemphasized?

✔ Is the curve in your low back too deep, forcing your belly to hang out?

✔ Are your shoulders sort of rolled over to the front, forcing your chest to sink in?

✔ Are your head and chin protruding to the front so that if you dropped a line from your ear lobe to the floor the line would fall in front of your chest?

Straightening and relaxing into the T'ai Chi Posture

Now you're ready for the "Infinite Ultimate." Hold on . . . what? Yes, indeedy, the basic T'ai Chi Posture, or Wu Chi stance, may be called just that: the Infinite Ultimate. That's because unless you stand well, you'll never move well, and if you can't move well, you'll never feel the chi.

This is not just about standing upright, but standing upright with power, without tension, and while being fully in control.

I'll describe the basic posture or stance to you, starting from the feet:

1. **Stand upright with your feet about shoulder-width apart, or perhaps 4–8 inches between them, and parallel.**

2. **Bend your knees slightly so they are not locked. Think of softening the joint.**

3. **Allow your tailbone to tuck under a little with the bend of the knees.**

   Don't force it. Your tailbone just drops under you slightly when you soften the knee joint. The curve in your *lumbar spine* (or low back) will flatten a little.

   Your body from the waist up has not been affected by anything you've done so far, has it? Good. Move on to the upper body.

4. **Relax your chest and shoulders.**

   That doesn't mean slouch, mind you. Just let the breath-holding military stance soften.

5. **Let your chest sink slightly.**

   Again, that doesn't mean turning into the Hunchback of Notre Dame, but rather just allow the chest to soften downward and slightly concave as a result of the shoulders relaxing.

6. **Feel your arms hanging naturally at your sides.**

7. **Imagine that your head is suspended above your body, as if a string is attached to the crown and pulling it upward. Feel the neck get longer and release.**

8. **Open your lips oh so slightly, as if you were starting to smile.**

9. **Touch your teeth lightly together, and let your tongue touch the upper palette just behind the front teeth.**

   This is said to help regulate the flow of saliva during practice.

    Don't clench your teeth! That'll bring more strain into your entire body!

10. **Finally, let all your muscles relax, breathe fully (I discuss breathing next), and let your gaze "go inward" so you are looking straight ahead while looking at nothing in particular.**

You are now in the Infinite Ultimate stance or a grand T'ai Chi Posture (see Figure 8-1). If a string with a small weight were dropped from the crown of your head, it would fall straight through your torso, down the middle of your pelvis, and land at a spot right between your feet.

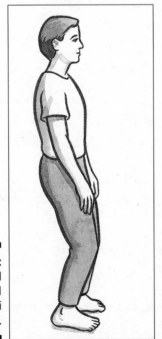

Figure 8-1:
Powerful
but relaxed
T'ai Chi
Posture.

T'ai Chi breathing

Breathing is a natural. You can stop on purpose, but not for long. And breath will be the last thing that leaves your body. But breathing fully isn't so natural. Getting locked up and breathing shallowly is easy with tension and stress — or just from sucking in those darn abs all the time.

Full and proper breathing is essential to developing your T'ai Chi practice.

T'ai Chi breathing is:

 ✔ Slow, just like the movements are slow.

 ✔ Full, but never forced.

 ✔ Coordinated with the movements for great flow.

Using your belly to breathe

T'ai Chi breathing uses the abdominals, not the chest. When you come into the world as a hollering newborn, you bellow using your abdominals, knowing full well that doing so will get you the most power — and will attract the most attention from mom or dad. As you grow up, you develop the habit of blocking your breath from reaching down into your abdominals, which doesn't use all of the lung's capacity — and certainly doesn't give you as much power either.

So, back to the abs you go.

A healthy, deep, full and powerful breath in, or inhalation, moves all the way down to your abdominal area (your belly, in laymen's terms!) and expands it outward. If you pumped up a balloon, it wouldn't stay flat, would it? Neither should your belly. When your belly expands, more air can get into your lungs. That also means more good oxygen goes into your blood, while more bad carbon dioxide gets pumped back out.

Don't force these deep breaths by sucking in or expanding more than you can naturally. And definitely don't let your shoulders hike up to try to get more air in.

When you exhale, or breathe out, the belly relaxes and simply lets the air escape back out. Just like you don't want to stop the inhalation before it gets to your abdominals, you also don't want to stop the exhalation before it fully releases the air in your lungs. But you also don't want to try to squeeze out any extra that doesn't flow out naturally.

When breathing in, try to center your breathing around the Dan Tien. (Take a look at Chapter 13 for more about this.) When breathing out, imagine energy flowing from the Dan Tien, up your spine, out to your hands and down your legs, and into your feet.

Imagine a wave moving through your body on each inhalation and exhalation. The wave flows the entire length of your torso from shoulders to pubic bone.

Coordinating your breath with your moves

To breathe in the T'ai Chi way, you have to do more than breathe with your belly. You also have to breathe in or out at the correct time with the movements. That will give you more power when you need it and more relaxation when you need that.

If you take a class somewhere, you may have a teacher who doesn't talk about the pattern of breathing until you've learned the movements. Others get right into breathing from Day 1 because they think it helps to develop slowness and softness in the movements.

You should know that there are different schools of thought on how to breathe — whether the abdomen should go in or go out on the inhale — well as whether to think about it at all. My simplistic opinion: Just remember to keep your breath moving in the way it feels best to you. Think about the mechanics later (if you even want to).

Here are four basic breathing guidelines:

- ✔ When you raise your arms, breathe in; when you lower your arms, breathe out.
- ✔ When you open your arms, breathe in; when you close your arms, breathe out.
- ✔ When you push out, breathe out; when you pull in, breathe in.
- ✔ When you strike (hands or feet), breathe out; when you withdraw, breathe in.

Really, don't think too hard about this breathing stuff and get yourself tense and tied up in knots. It is really very much common sense. Just let the body do what feels natural, then think about it. In most cases, you'll already be practicing the right pattern.

Bottom line: Don't stop breathing. Holding your breath is worse than breathing "wrong."

Putting on the Moves

After you conquer standing well and breathing well (shoot, this is like being a toddler again!), you finally get to move your body a little. But you're still not running, only walking.

THERESE'S TWO CENTS

Un-graining old habits

Like anyone else learning T'ai Chi, you may have experience in some other movement form, be it dance, a combat martial art, running, or something else. Those ingrained habits may affect your learning curve as you take on the basics of holding your hands and moving your feet.

I for one have done my share of various dance forms, and my hands immediately want to turn into a ballet dancer's with slightly soft wrists and a middle finger that hangs down a little. T'ai Chi teachers point it out, and I try to change, then the old habits take over again. So don't get impatient with yourself. All of this takes time.

Some instructors won't break apart the positions of the feet or hands and teach them separately from the forms themselves. Maybe it's my Western mind, but I want to know what one part looks like so I can do it right after I start moving. So here they are, the basic hand and feet positions, as well as a couple of transitions that will come up repeatedly.

Understanding directions

Typically, in classical T'ai Chi, you find that the movement is oriented in two ways: by compass (north, south, east, west) or by clockface (12 o'clock, 6 o'clock, and so on). That takes some thinking compared to traditional Western exercise where you just face front, wherever front is, then turn right or turn left.

There are different schools of thought as to which method is better. When you use the face of a clock (as I do in this book) your front — wherever that may be — becomes 12 o'clock. (Okay, in *most* cases the front becomes 12 o'clock. Here comes another exception: Some call the *rear* true 12 o'clock. *Remember:* Nothing is truly wrong if there is a reason for it, and it's consistent.) For you, if your front is 12, then your right is 3, to the rear is 6, and to your left is 9. I like this better because 12 is then 12. Period.

On the other hand, when you use a compass, you may hear an instructor say, "Face north," but that doesn't necessarily mean true polar north. North may just be a representation of wherever the front happens to be. As a navigational sort, I find this method sort of boggling to my senses. The other way of figuring out which way is which is to simply call the positions front, back, right, and left. Unfortunately, with T'ai Chi's minute shifts, that can be very inexact. Does 2 o'clock (or northeast) become front-right? Take a look at Figure 8-2 so you can see how all this fits together.

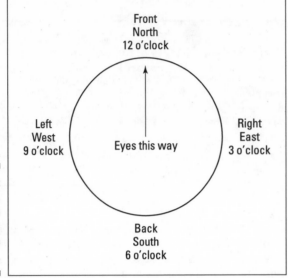

Figure 8-2:
Following
the T'ai Chi
map and
compass
for forms.

My collaborator Manny, who uses directions, throws a different light on all this, and we had some fun talking to each other about forms in these different directional "languages." He points out that there is really a different "clock-face" for both the body (with the spine being the middle point about which the hands and torso move) and for the foot (with the heel being the middle point). You will note when you get to the basics later in this chapter, as well as the forms in Chapters 8 through 11, that I will, at times, say your torso faces X o'clock, but your toes face X o'clock.

Handling your hands and arms

Take a few moments to review these static positions. If you see — and feel them — in isolation, you can improve a movement or position after you set it in motion. Of course, you get to see illustrations along the way too so you can look and mimic if that suits your learning style better.

T'ai Chi Arm and Hand

The goal for your arms and hands is to remain curved and soft, but still full of energy and exuding some power, rather than being limp. You do *not* bring your middle finger in a little, as ballet dancers do (and I have a habit of doing). The whole point of this curved yet strong position is to help the flow of chi through your body and up and down your limbs. See Figure 8-3 for an illustration of how to hold your arms and hands.

1. **Hold both arms straight out in front of your shoulders, palms facing in, with fingers, hands and elbows straight.**

2. **Let your fingers and thumbs soften slightly so your palm develops a slight cup, as if you were trying to hold onto a medium-sized ball with just one hand. Your fingers relax apart but aren't forced.**

3. **At the same time, allow your elbows to soften and widen outward slightly (something they want to do automatically when you soften your hands). The elbows don't sag downward, though.**

4. **Now imagine holding one very, very large ball between your hands. Move that ball up and down in front of you without altering the position of your hands.**

You now have one smooth curved line from your shoulder, around the outside of your elbow and down the back of your wrist and hand to the end of your fingers. Remember that curves are a key principle of T'ai Chi. Refer to Chapter 7 for more on the principles. Your wrist is soft, but not bent in so much that you have an abrupt change in angle between your forearm and back of your hand. Any abrupt angle can put a kink in your chi hose.

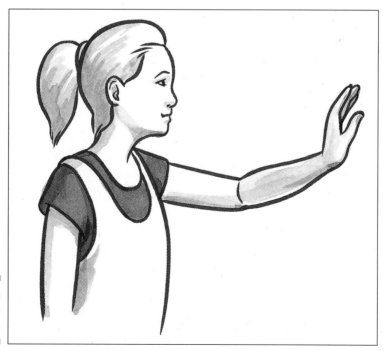

Figure 8-3:
T'ai Chi Arm
and Hand.

If you held your smooth and curved T'ai Chi Arm and Hand with the palm down, imagine that a bead of water could roll from the elbow right off the back of your palm.

Hold Balloon

The names for the Hold Balloon hand position (also called Holding the Ball or Embracing the Moon) are inspired by what it looks and feels like. I have a soft spot for the name Hold Balloon because it feels lighter, softer, and floatier to me.

In this position, you feel as if you are holding a balloon (great deduction, Sherlock) in front of your body. Your arms and hands on the top and bottom look and feel as if they are conforming to the circle of a very large inflated balloon. See Figure 8-4.

Start standing in a feet-parallel stance so you don't have to think about what the feet are up to. After you have the Hold Balloon down, you can try it with other steps too. One step where it comes up often is in the Centering Step that you can read about where I introduce transitions, later in this chapter.

1. **Bring your left hand, palm up, and your arm across your body at the level of your hips, but don't extend your left hand beyond your right side.**

2. **Bring your right hand, palm down, and your arm across your body at the level of your chest, but don't extend it beyond your left side.**

3. **Soften both elbows and remember to practice basic T'ai Chi Arm and Hand! You are now holding a balloon between your arms and hands.**

4. **Try the same position with the opposite hand on top because you will be switching sides frequently in the forms.**

The hand positions and levels change slightly based on the form you are going into or coming out of, as do they also change a bit depending on a teacher's style or school.

T'ai Chi Fist

The style of T'ai Chi fist that I use in this book is a vertical fist. In other words, if you opened your hand while in the fist, you'd look like you were about to shake hands with someone instead of whack them in the gut. This puts the bones of the forearm and hand in a stronger and more stabile position, like that shown in Figure 8-5. Other schools use different types of fists.

1. **Hold your hand in front of you as if you wanted to shake hands with someone.**

2. **Close the fingers to make a fist with the thumb resting on top of the knuckles toward the center of your body, not tucked up inside of the fingers. The fist is closed fully but not squeezed shut.**

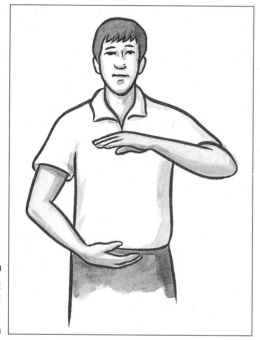

Figure 8-4:
Hold
Balloon.

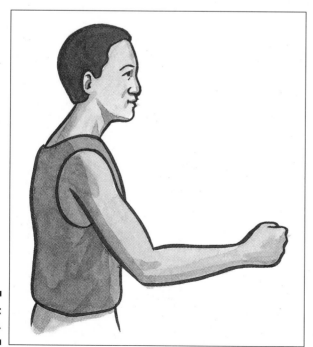

Figure 8-5:
T'ai Chi Fist.

The wrist is not cocked backward because that is weak. Instead, make sure the back of the hand is basically on one plane with the top of your forearm.

Compared to Western fist-dom, the muscles in the forearm and hand stay relaxed. No need to expend extra energy just making the fist!

Dropped Hand

The Dropped Hand, also called Hook Hand or Beak Hand, is one hand position that just screams T'ai Chi. In the Yang Short Form introduced in Chapters 9 through 11, the Dropped Hand only appears in the Single Whip form. But it's unusual enough — and can reappear in other forms if you do more T'ai Chi — that I think it's worth illustrating on its own.

The hardest part of this can be doing the Dropped Hand with one hand, while the other hand stays relaxed. It'll feel at first like rubbing your stomach and patting your head! See Figure 8-6 for an illustration of the Dropped Hand.

1. **Hold one arm out to your side, palm down.**

2. **Pull your fingers down and together, placing the tips of your thumb and fingers (except your little finger) together. Your little finger tucks in between the ring finger and thumb.**

3. **Allow your knuckles to soften just a tiny bit so your hand, if you pulled it up so the fingers pointed straight out, indeed would like the beak of a goose. Just like in the Fist, the fingers and forearm stay relaxed, not tense.**

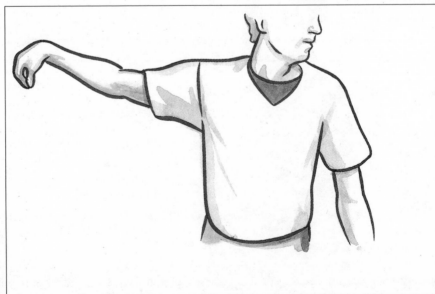

Figure 8-6:
Dropped
Hand.

It feels as if you were trying to pick up a really small object from a tabletop. If you did actually put your fingers down on a level surface, they would all (except the little guy on the end by some people) actually touch the surface.

You may actually feel as if you were getting ready to play shadow games on your wall, with a goose being the first one to dance across the light!

Footing the basics

Because you're on your feet, the stances that your feet make are an important part of T'ai Chi. In fact, they can make or break your practice. Unless you've got the feet positioned well, you can lose chi (that's that energy flow again) and therefore power. If you aren't looking for a fight (and you probably aren't), what you'll be losing is your ability to relax and feel the peace and tranquility that a good energy flow can bring.

Two stances — Bow Stance and Empty Step — come up again and again in the short form covered in Chapters 9 through 11. I also introduce two others, however — Single Leg and Riding the Horse — that are good to practice because of the balance (or meditative power) and the leg strength they bring. If you do more than just dabble in T'ai Chi, these two will be key skills.

Bow Stance

Practice the Bow Stance (also called the Bow and Arrow Step or Arched Step) 'til you're blue in the face because it's the foundation of many T'ai Chi movements. The reason for the name is that you bend your front leg a bit like a primed bow, and your back leg is straighter, like an arrow ready for flight. Now that's just figurative because your back leg isn't really straight, but you still get the bow-and-arrow analogy to help you remember what the stance looks like. You can see the position in Figure 8-7. It is not as symmetrical as other stances so the challenges will be greater to your muscles. You can also practice the Bow with various hand positions and hold it for a meditation, too.

1. **Start standing with both feet parallel and about hip-width apart, facing 12 o'clock. Bend your knees slightly, keeping your weight centered over your feet and your hips tucked under slightly. See T'ai Chi posture for all the reminders.**

   This feet-parallel stance is a typical stance for starting and closing forms, as well as a stance for meditation.

2. **Turn your right foot out slightly (about 45 degrees or to about halfway between 1 and 2 o'clock, or to 1:30) by pivoting on your heel to point your toes outward.**

   This allows you to keep your hips dropped and your spine aligned and not forced into a swayback position. Shift your weight onto your left foot slightly before you put the weight back onto your right foot.

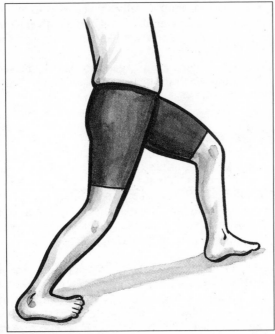

Figure 8-7:
Bow
Stance.

3. **Nearly at the same time you're pivoting on your heel, begin bending your right knee slightly and shifting your weight onto your right foot. At the same time, raise your left knee, lifting your left toe off the ground, and step out to the front leading with your heel. Land first (and softly!) onto the floor with your heel, rolling the rest of your foot down flat.**

Imagine that you're trying to sneak up on somebody and you want to be really, really quiet!

4. **As your left foot lands, your right leg nearly straightens, pushing about 60–70 percent of your weight onto your front leg, which is bending at the knee. Your stance now looks like a lunge.**

When you get into the position, make sure that your left toes point directly forward. The toes on your right foot should point outward slightly. Plus, you should have some width between your feet (about shoulder-width) — as if your heels were placed on opposite corners of a square on the ground.

Empty Step

This step gets its name because your rear foot is *full* (carrying 100 percent of your weight), while your front foot is *empty* (carrying none of your weight). The yin-yang concept of opposites mixing to provide a perfect balance comes into play here.

The Empty Step, as you can see in Figure 8-8, is in some ways another transitional step that you don't usually start from a simple standing position. But use these step-by-step instructions to get into a correct position so you can feel and practice it while stationary before putting it into motion.

Empty Step is a lot like the Centering Step (see "Centering Step" in the next section on Transitions) except the hip of your non-weight-bearing "empty" foot is turned in and that toe is in front of the supporting leg, not beside it. Note that I present this step with the entire foot of the front "empty" foot on the ground. Some teachers will do the heel of the front foot lifted so just the toe or ball of the foot is on the ground. You may even see it with the heel on the ground instead. You need an open mind to all the teaching styles, as always.

1. **Start standing with both feet parallel and about hip-width apart. Bend your knees slightly, keeping your weight centered over your feet and your hips tucked under slightly. Position your toes as if you are toeing an imaginary straight line on the ground in front of you.**

2. **Step directly forward with your left foot, placing your heel on the other side of the imaginary line.**

3. **Shift your weight backward, bending both knees as deeply as you can.**

   You should be balanced and rooted on your right leg strongly enough that you can lift the front left heel, toe, or the entire foot off the ground and not fall or be forced to shift your body position.

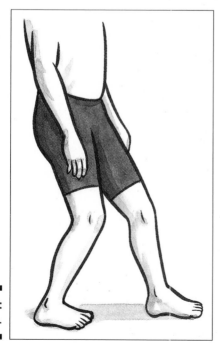

Figure 8-8:
Empty Step.

To help you really feel the weight shift, try rocking this step forward and backward slowly and gently from front foot to rear foot. Just transfer most of your weight onto the front foot, rock it all backward onto the rear foot (taking a moment to find your balance), and then lift your front foot slightly. Be sure to alternate the foot you put forward — one side of your body is always stronger than the other.

Single Leg Stance

Although not a transitional step or one that comes up in nearly ever move like the Bow Stance, this step requires enough practice that perfecting it while stationary can help you flow through it later. See Figure 8-9 for an illustration.

1. **Stand with both feet parallel and about hip-width apart, facing 12 o'clock. Bend your knees slightly, keeping your weight centered over your feet. You can just let your arms hang at your side.**

   Be sure to engage strong and centered T'ai Chi Posture in this standing position before you try to move on. If you don't, you'll teeter and maybe even fall over as you actually lift one leg.

2. **Shift just a little bit more of your weight over your right foot.**

3. **Gradually lift your left knee until the thigh is parallel to the floor, or as high as you can get it. Avoid wobbling too!**

4. **Stay there a moment and then lower the foot slowly down, placing it softly back into its original position.**

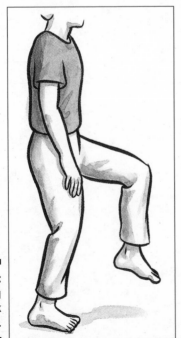

Figure 8-9:
Standing like a stork on one leg.

Be sure to do this balance-testing and balance-honing stance on both sides. Everybody is better on one side. When you figure out your least-skilled side, do that one more.

Riding the Horse

Despite being used more often as a training and leg-strengthening position, Riding the Horse (also called T'ai Chi Stance or Riding the Goat) is a basic posture you want to let your body feel. You can use it as a meditation position after your legs are strong enough in it.

When you first try this, keep your feet only slightly wider than your shoulders. As you get stronger, they can move out wider and wider, which is of course more and more challenging to the muscles in your legs and buttocks! See Figure 8-10.

1. **Start in Wu Chi or basic T'ai Chi Posture. (See Figure 8-1 earlier in this chapter.)**

2. **Shift your weight slightly onto your right foot and step out with your left foot so the stance's width becomes just slightly wider than your shoulders.**

3. **Place the foot back on the floor. Let your knees bend, but tighten your buttocks muscles to keep your knees rotated out toward your feet, rather than rolling inward. Sink into the stance. You will feel as if you are indeed astride a horse.**

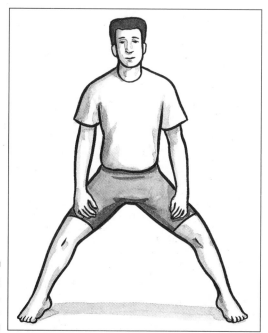

Figure 8-10:
Giddy-up, little pony.

Focus on keeping your tailbone slightly tucked under. If you try to go wider or sink lower than your flexibility or strength can, you'll probably end up sticking your butt out behind with a swayback.

At all costs, avoid letting your knees flop or buckle inward so the joint is hanging out with nothing but open air between it and the ground. That can strain the knee joint. If you can't keep the knees open, then narrow the stance.

Stepping into transitions

If you read Chapter 7 on T'ai Chi principles, you may remember the section on flow. One of the beauties — and one of the challenges — of good T'ai Chi is flowing all the movements, both hand and feet, so there is really no stop, no period, no hiccup. That's where good transitions come in — to help you keep the flow, especially as a novice.

Centering Step

This transitional step merely lets you shift your weight from one side to the other. But to do it well is a moment of pure heaven when you feel as if you are floating above the ground and totally in control of your body's movement. Developing balance is what gets you to that nanosecond of bliss.

You don't normally just stand around in the Centering Step (also called the T-Step), as shown in Figure 8-11, but use it to move into other positions. Throughout the Yang Short Form in Chapters 9 through 11 and in Manny's Short Form in Chapter 12, you come across Centering Steps sprinkled here and there. In most cases, after you have really good balance, you can ignore this step and simply float the foot through and into the next position.

So use this drill to practice your body positioning and balance.

1. **Stand with both feet parallel and about hip-width apart. Bend your knees slightly (just soften the joint), keeping your weight centered over your feet and your tailbone tucked under slightly.**

2. **Shift your hips (and your body weight) from a centered position over both feet to a centered position over your right foot, bending your right knee a little more.**

3. **At the same time, lift your left foot and bring the base of your toes onto the ground next to the arch of your right foot.**

4. **Open out your left knee and hip slightly, using the muscles in your buttocks and hips to rotate the knee outward.**

This is an open Qua position. Take a look at the sidebar on Qua (pronounced *kwa* and sometimes spelled differently) in this section to get the hang of what this Qua stuff is all about.

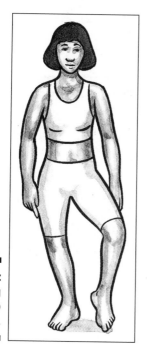

Figure 8-11:
Stepping
into
Centering.

You should be able to stand in this balanced position with no weight on your lifted knee. Try to lift that toe for a moment — you should be able to do this without falling over.

Sweep Open Step

Some of these transitions aren't real steps in and unto themselves. This one (and the next one, the Bow-to-Empty Step) are both of this type. I plucked these two steps out of the 24-movement form because they come up a few times. Once again, learn them in isolation so you can recognize them in the forms and already know what to do.

Take a look at Figure 8-12 for a look at this move. Like the Centering Step, it is used to simply get you to the other side. You'll see it, for example, to move you between Grasp the Bird's Tail on the left, and Grasp the Bird's Tail on the right, which are the last two forms in Chapter 9.

I call it "Sweep Open" because, as you see, you sort of sweep your arms and body open to the front during the step.

JARGON ALERT

Conquering Your Qua

Qua (pronounced *kwa*) refers to the area of the body across the front of what Westerners call the pelvis. Opening the qua is done by keeping the knees and feet open rather than turned in toward one another. If you've ever studied any dance, such as ballet, it's a bit like a turned-out position through the hips. In T'ai Chi practice, the qua remains open — always. Physically, an open qua allows the tailbone to tuck under more easily (as I described in the section on T'ai Chi Posture, earlier in this chapter). Energetically, it also keeps the back straight, which helps the chi channels up and down your back stay open so the chi can get to and from where it needs to go. Standing meditation is excellent for learning to keep the qua open, but it does require some strength and flexibility in muscles and ligaments not often challenged in the West. So, as always, patience is recommended, especially as you learn to become aware of the qua.

1. **Start standing in a Bow Stance with your left foot forward (see Figure 8-7) facing 9 o'clock. For this practice, leave your arms at your sides.**

2. **Shift your weight onto your right foot, keeping the knee bent. Now, "sweep open" or rotate your body fully to face the front or 12 o'clock. The left leg extends but the knee joint doesn't lock, and your left foot rotates in so the left toes also face 12 o'clock by pivoting on the heel.**

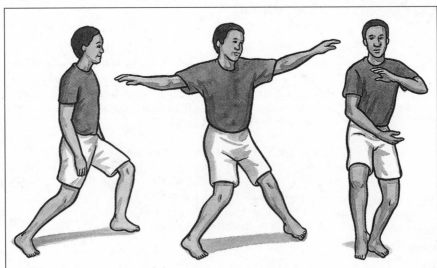

Figure 8-12:
Sweep
Open Step.

3. **At the same time as you rotate the body open, float both arms up and out to each side, palms facing down. You may feel like a bird ready for flight.**

4. **To finish, shift your weight back to your left foot. Draw your right toes in to a Centering Step (see Figure 8-11) over your left foot, with your arms to a Hold Balloon position (see Figure 8-4) with the left arm on top.**

Bow-to-Empty Step

Okay, I just made up this name too because I had to call it something when I plucked it out of the form to teach you separately! See Figure 8-13 for an illustration to guide you. When you read it as part of the instruction for a form in Chapters 9 through 12, you'll know to turn back here for more detail. The first time it comes up is at the beginning of the form White Crane Cools Its Wings, the third form of the Yang Short Form presented in Chapter 9.

As with the Sweep Open Step or the Centering Step, use this step to get you smoothly from one position or direction to another position or direction.

I called this "Bow-to-Empty" because you use this to shift from the Bow Stance to an Empty Step.

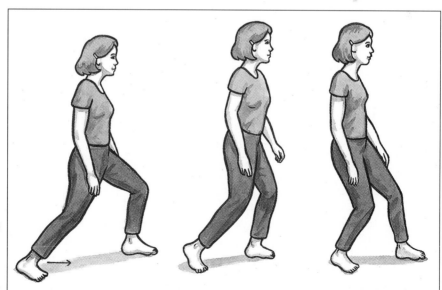

Figure 8-13:
Bow-to-
Empty Step.

1. **Start standing in a Bow Stance with your left foot forward (see Figure 8-7) facing 9 o'clock.**

2. **Let your weight rock forward onto your left foot to release your right foot.**

3. **Then step in softly with your right foot about a half-step closer to your left. Now let your weight rock backward onto the right foot, letting your front left foot become "empty" or unweighted so you are now in an Empty Step.**

Letting Yourself Move

Basics aren't just standing still or transitioning your positions. They're also about learning to move, gradually of course, baby step by baby step. Part of that means putting a few things together. Part of it also means knowing how to warm-up your body. So I move into those areas next on your safari through the land of basics.

Warming up

T'ai Chi is, of course, performed quite slowly, as you read in Chapter 7 about the principles. So, you may ask, why do you need to warm-up before an activity like T'ai Chi that is slow enough to be a warm-up all by itself?

Well, you may *not* need to:

- As you get more advanced and get to know your own body's needs better.
- When you are doing simple meditative stances that involve little or no movement.
- If you do other activity before you do T'ai Chi so you're already warmed up.

But many people, and perhaps you too, will indeed need to warm up, especially if you are:

- A beginner at any kind of exercise.
- Rehabilitating from an injury or strain, or if you suffer from some kind of pain such as low-back problems or arthritis.
- Need to help your mind "warm-up" and focus as much as your body.

T'ai Chi, no matter how slow, still challenges the leg, knees, and hips. You can get sore, even if you are very fit from other activities. A little bit of warm-up can help you feel better when you do start and definitely feel better afterward or even the next day.

Physiologically, a warm-up for any movement:

- ✔ Loosens the muscles and joints so you can move more easily and with more flexibility, which can reduce the chance of strain and injury.

- ✔ Raises the core body temperature (why do you think they call it a "warm-up?") so your muscles are softer — like taffy that's been in the sun.

- ✔ Shifts how your body uses oxygen so oxygen leaving the bloodstream can more readily get into and help out working muscles.

To warm-up, you can do other activities, move through forms and stances much more easily with less bend in the knees but perhaps a bit faster so you feel warmer, or do a few loosening exercises that target areas T'ai Chi will use. Manny uses the warm-up movements below. You can too.

Beyond just warming up your muscles and joints, a warm-up session can give you a few minutes to quiet yourself and your mind. You prepare yourself to practice your forms — externally *and* internally — with more focus. You can use this time to center your energy, forget any upset, start breathing fully, or release any tension — or even just to find the tension you need to release.

Repeat each warm-up movement for 30–60 seconds each, for a total of 5–10 minutes of warming up. After you've tried them all, you may find one doesn't feel comfortable or even necessary. If so, leave that one out. Feel free to add some other movement that you feel you need instead.

Do these in the order presented.

Flop Twists

Try these easy twisting motions when you start as a way to shake out your muscles and to make sure your feet are rooted. Like the name says, just let yourself flop about like a Raggedy Ann doll.

1. **Stand with your feet parallel and about shoulder-width apart, with your knees slightly bent. Your arms are hanging at your sides.**

2. **Swing your body easily, without any force, from side-to-side, letting your arms flop with your body. Your arms may even kind of whack you on each side or as high as your chest as they swing about like cooked spaghetti. Be sure you continue to breathe throughout.**

3. **Continue to look straight ahead as your body swings.**

If you have a bad back, or have had any back injuries, consult with your physician before trying this warm-up. If you get the go-ahead to practice, keep the swings smaller and more controlled.

Flop Arms

In this warm-up, you may feel as if you're paddling along on an air mattress belly-down or legs-down through the middle of an inner tube — and getting nowhere fast! You're still flopping about loosely.

1. **Stand with your feet parallel and about shoulder-width apart, with your knees slightly bent. Your arms are hanging at your sides.**

2. **Raise your arms up to about shoulder-height in front of you, keeping the curve described in T'ai Chi Arm and Hand (see Figure 8-3 earlier in this chapter).**

3. **Let your arms swing back with a big push, as if you're paddling yourself through water. They only go as far as feels natural.**

4. **Let your arms flop back to the front in a passive return from the momentum of your back swing, again letting the arms only return as far as they move naturally. Continue to breathe fully and naturally.**

I Dunno Shoulders

The movements in this warm-up may make you feel as if you're repeatedly saying, "I dunno." But you do know what you're doing — you're warming up your shoulders. See Figure 8-14.

1. **Stand with your feet parallel and about shoulder-width apart, with your knees slightly bent. Let your arms hang loosely from your shoulders. Your arms play no part in this warm-up!**

2. **Inhale and lift one shoulder as high toward your ear as you can, then let it drop with a full exhalation.**

3. **Inhale and lift the opposite shoulder as high toward your ear as you can, then let it drop down with a big exhalation.**

4. **Repeat the individual shoulders 8–10 times each, then start the I Dunno pattern. See Step 5.**

5. **Lift both shoulders at the same time as you inhale hold and tense, then drop and feel utter relaxation with a full exhalation.**

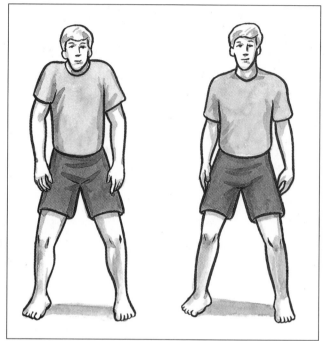

Figure 8-14:
I Dunno
Shoulders…
so you
know.

Circling Shoulders

Because you circle your shoulders and use that joint a lot in T'ai Chi, warming up that motion can be helpful too.

1. **Stand with your feet parallel and about shoulder-width apart, with your knees slightly bent. Let your arms hang loosely from your shoulders. Do one I Dunno shoulder lift (both shoulders) and hold it for a split second. Inhale with this movement.**

2. **With both shoulders still lifted toward your ears, rotate both shoulders backward and then start to pull them downward, feeling the stretch across your chest. Begin to exhale.**

3. **Then drop your shoulders all the way down as if you were holding heavy buckets full of wet sand in each hand.**

4. **Finish by pulling your shoulders forward as if you were cold and trying to cower a bit. Finish your exhale, inhale once, exhale again, and then start the whole pattern again.**

5. **Repeat 10–12 times, focusing on opening your chest and releasing any tension in your shoulders. Use the breath to help you.**

Neck Circles

Anytime you circle the neck, you need to be very careful. You never drop the weight of your head back and crunch your spine in your neck. See Figure 8-15.

If you have or ever have had any neck, head, or upper back injuries, you should consult a physician before trying this. And take these out of your repertoire if they ever hurt at all!

1. **Stand with your feet parallel and about shoulder-width apart, with your knees slightly bent. Let your arms hang loosely from your shoulders, or place your hands on your waist.**

2. **While continuing to look straight ahead with your eyes, circle your neck in one direction about 10 times. Then circle in the other direction.**

Don't twist your neck or try to look down, up, or over your shoulder. If you stood a mirror in front of you, you should be able to look yourself in the eyes the entire time.

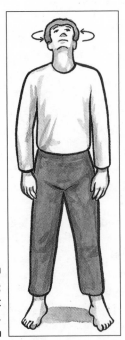

Figure 8-15:
Circle that
neck.

Torso Circles

A little waist movement can help warm you up for the turning in T'ai Chi too. See Figure 8-16.

1. **Stand with your feet parallel and about shoulder-width apart, with your knees slightly bent. Place your hands on your waist, and tip your upper body forward just a teeny bit.**

2. **Just like with neck circles, you continue to face straight ahead with your head and torso. Rotate your upper body from the waist about 5–8 times going in one direction, then repeat on the other side.**

3. **When that is comfortable, you can add about 5 rotations to each side with your arms at your side instead of on your waist.**

Don't twist your body. When you learn forward, feel your low back stretch or pull just a little. When you lean backward, feel your waist or abdominal muscles stretch just a little.

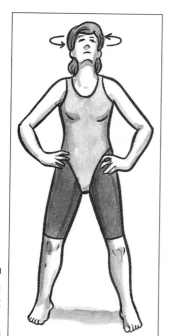

Figure 8-16:
Circle that torso.

Swimming

You're still loosening up your shoulders with this one, this time with full rotations around your body though.

1. **Stand with feet a little wider than shoulder-width apart with your hands on your hips, and your knees slightly bent.**

2. **Begin to mimic a forward stroke in swimming with your arms: Bring your right arm down and back, then over your head to the front. When the right arm is to the front, add the left going backward, then over your head to the front. One arm is to the front when one is to the back.**

3. **Let your body turn slightly forward with the forward arm as if you want to reach farther.**

4. **Repeat about 15 times going forward, then do the backstroke by reversing the rotation.**

Hula Hips

You may want to make sure you're the only one in the room when you try this hip-loosening exercise!

1. **Stand with feet a little wider than shoulder-width apart with your hands on your hips.**

2. **Bend your knees a little and swing your hips slowly in a full circle as if you are trying to keep a hula hoop up (only you'd be going faster if you really were).**

3. **Repeat about 10–15 times in each direction. Make sure you keep the breath moving in and out throughout.**

Drawing Circles with Your Toes

When you do this exercise, you should feel as if you're trying to draw a big circle in front of you in the air with your big toe.

1. **Stand on one foot, holding onto the wall or a chair as needed for balance.**

2. **Draw big imaginary circles in the air with the toes of the foot you're not standing on 8–10 times in each direction.**

3. **Change feet and repeat. Be sure not to hold your breath!**

Drawing Circles with Your Knees

You want to stay nice and loose in your body for this one. No tensing or forcing the circles.

1. **Stand with the right foot slightly more forward than the left foot with both knees bent. There is only a little weight on the forward foot — only enough for you to keep your balance — and the entire foot touches the floor.**

2. **Rotate your knee in space, as if you are trying to draw a circle parallel to the ground with your kneecap. The movement actually comes from your hip; it just comes out looking like a knee circle.**

3. **Repeat for 8–10 circles, reverse direction, and then switch sides and do both directions on the left.**

Lunging Side-to-Side

You can do this one with knees bent more or less, depending on your strength and flexibility. Take a look at Figure 8-17 for some idea what it looks like.

Avoid leaning over to the point where you feel any strain in your back (no more lean than Figure 8-17 shows). Also, don't do it if you know you have a bad back.

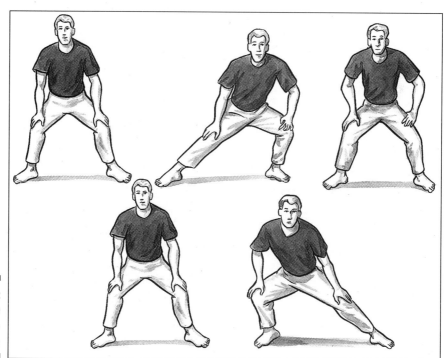

Figure 8-17:
Side to
side . . .
that's right.

1. **Stand with your feet about a foot or two wider than shoulder-width apart. Turn out your toes slightly (about 45 degrees). Bend your knees and lean over just a little so you can put your hands on your thighs. You may feel like a football quarterback getting right for a hike.**

   You will use your hands on your thighs to support your body weight when you start moving your body weight side-to-side in the lunge.

2. **Shift your body weight to your right side, letting your left knee straighten.**

3. **Now move to the left side (stay as low as you can!) by bending your left knee and sliding your weight across the center of your stance to the left side. The right knee straightens when you reach the left side.**

4. **Return to standing with your weight coming over the center and your hands releasing from your thighs as your legs straighten.**

5. **Repeat by leaning over and starting the body-weight shift to the left. Repeat 3–4 times per side.**

Doing your T'ai Chi scales

T'ai Chi practitioners don't do a lot of drills as a part of their practice. Some of that is because of time demands — why spend it doing drills when you can get down to business? — and part of it is because of tradition — just do it, so to speak.

I look at a drill as "T'ai Chi scales." When you learn the piano, you don't start out by doing Beethoven's 5th, even if you go slowly and note by note. You start with little drills and practices so you become nimble enough to tackle Mozart, perhaps even later in your same lesson in some small part.

When you first try some T'ai Chi, you also may need a little practice, like doing your scales. This drill, conceived by my collaborator Manny, won't always be a part of your practice. At first, it may be all of it. Later, you may do some of this as a short session on its own, or just for a kind of warm-up before you start doing the forms. Finally, you may not do it at all. Then again, you may be the kind of person who even at the beginning wants to cut straight to the quick, and that's fine too! Do what feels best to you — always. This is here as yet another piece of the menu from which you can choose.

If you do choose to try this drill, focus not only on the physical movement, but also on the connection with your energy as well as on all the basics in this chapter about positioning and in Chapter 7 on the key principles of T'ai Chi.

Chapters 17 through 19 present other combinations and forms you can do to make the most of your practice as it develops. Take a look there for some ideas too.

Linking up the basics

Now you get to put a few basics together for your own practice form. Refer to earlier sections in this chapter for all the detailed instruction and figures.

1. **Wu Chi stance,** facing 12 o'clock

2. **Empty Step** four times, moving forward (left foot, then right, left, and finish with right forward)

3. **Bow Stance, left**

4. **Bow Stance, right** — turn 90 degrees to the right to face 3 o'clock

5. **Bow Stance, left** — turn back 90 degrees to the left to face 12 o'clock

6. **Centering Step** with Hold Balloon, left arm on top

7. **Bow Stance, right**

8. **Bow Stance, left** — turn 90 degrees to the left to face 9 o'clock

9. **Bow Stance, right** — turn back 90 degrees to the right to face 12 o'clock

10. **Centering Step** with Hold Balloon, left arm on top

11. **Empty Step** four times, moving backward (right foot, then left, right, and finish with left stepping back)

12. **Wu Chi stance,** facing 12 o'clock

13. **Riding the Horse stance**

Working through the drill

In the previous section, I list the names in order of what you do in the drill. Here is some additional instruction to help you through it.

1. **From the Wu Chi stance, shift your weight slowly to the left leg and turn your right foot out 45 degrees by lifting the toe to pivot on the heel. That puts the toes facing between 2 and 3 o'clock. Leave your arms at your side, practicing T'ai Chi hand.**

2. **Shift your weight back onto the right leg. Step your left foot forward into an Empty Step. Your left foot will be in front of your left hip without any weight placed over it. During this series of Empty Steps, if you like, you can lift your hands, so the palms face down at about hip-level, as if you were placing your hands on a table.**

   To make sure you are keeping the front foot in the Empty Step "empty" or unweighted, bring your left foot back beside the right in a Centering Step. If you have to push off from the left foot or move your body's position in space to do this, the left foot was not empty. Repeat this several times until it's truly empty.

3. **From the left foot forward Empty Step, turn your left foot out forty-five degrees (as always, by lifting the toe and pivoting on the heel).**

Shift your weight onto the left leg and step forward into an Empty Step with the right foot forward.

4. Step forward again with your left foot into another Empty step, as in Step 3. Finish the series by stepping forward with your right foot again into the last Empty Step. You will have moved forward just a little.

5. Turn your right foot out forty-five degrees (remember the toe-lifting and heel-pivoting?) and shift your weight forward onto the right leg.

6. Step forward with your left foot into a Bow Stance. You can, if you'd like, raise your arms from the shoulders, still maintaining good T'ai Chi curves in the elbow, and push forward with your palms.

Remember the Bow Stance is as wide as it is long, with the heels at opposite corners of an imaginary square. About 60–70 percent of your weight is over the front leg.

7. Shift your weight back onto the right leg, freeing your left foot to pivot on the heel 45 degrees to the *right* (inward). Shift your weight back onto the left leg as you turn your body 90 degrees to the right. You now face 3 o'clock. Step forward to 3 o'clock with your right foot into a Bow Stance. You can move your right foot through a Centering Step for practice or if you need the balance. Also, let your arms float from a push position, back to your sides.

8. Shift the weight back to the left leg to free the right foot. Turn the right foot to the *left* (inward) on the heel 45 degrees. Turn the body to face 12 o'clock again. Step forward to 12 o'clock with your left foot into a Bow Stance. Use a Centering Step on the way if you want to. Push forward with your palms again if you'd like.

Note the inward pivots of the feet in the last two moves. Practice those well because they too come up in the forms in Chapter 9 through 12.

9. Shift your weight back onto the right leg, freeing the left foot to pivot outward 45 degrees. Shift the weight onto the left leg. Step forward with your right foot into a Centering Step so the right toes graze the ground (or are "empty" so that they have no weight on them) next to the left ankle. Bring your arms into Hold Balloon with left arm on top.

10. Step forward into a Bow Stance to 12 o'clock with your right foot. You now repeat the same series of Bow Stances, as in Steps 7–8, except on the opposite side so you turn to the left or to 9 o'clock. Your first one will be with the left leg to 9 o'clock. Then you turn back to face 12 o'clock with the right leg forward.

11. Repeat the weight-shift backward as in Step 9, except you are shifting back onto your left leg. Then go into another Centering Step, the same as in Step 9 with your weight on your left leg, right toes grazing the ground and arms in Hold Balloon with left arm on top.

In a Centering Step, if the right foot is empty, then the accompanying Hold Balloon places the left arm on top. If the left foot is empty — guess what — the right arm is on top.

12. Now step the right foot *backward* (that's right, *backward*) into an Empty Step with the left foot finishing in front of you, empty of course. Repeat the steps moving backward so you have a series of four Empty Steps, finishing with the right foot forward. You can again place your hands at hip-height, palms facing down, as if they were on a table, if you'd like.

13. To finish, bring the right foot back under you into the Wu Chi stance. Shift your weight back equally over both feet. Straighten upward slightly and drop your arms and hands to your sides.

14. Finally, bend your knees again. Step your left foot out wide into a Ride the Horse Stance. Hold this final stance for as long as you can. Practice your T'ai Chi Posture and T'ai Chi Breathing. Place your hands in a comfortable position, such as at your side or palms down, as in Step 13.

Chapter 9

Opening the Door, Yang-Style

● ●

In This Chapter

▶ Getting to a short form from a much longer form

▶ Tackling the first eight forms in the flow

▶ Grasping the Bird's Tail is all about the principles

● ●

*T*here isn't really just one Yang form. Well, okay, there sort of used to be, but over the years, it's been added to, modified, and tweaked a bit by practitioners around the world to suit personal concepts of what worked best or felt best.

Rest easy, though. All the Yang Short Forms (also known as *Yang-style Short Form, Yang Simplified Form, Yang 24-Movement Short Form,* or *Yang Short Form*) you encounter are very similar, although some have as many as 37 movements compared to the 24-movement form that I present here. No form is wrong, just different. You end up discovering more through the challenges of experiencing different concepts.

The first portion of the Yang 24-movement form contains a heaping portion of the hallmark movements from the Yang long form. These forms, in the order they appear in this chapter, are

> Commencement or Opening the Door
>
> Parting the Wild Horse's Mane
>
> White Crane Cools its Wings
>
> Brush Knee
>
> Strum the Lute
>
> Repulse the Monkey
>
> Grasp the Bird's Tail — Left
>
> Grasp the Bird's Tail — Right

Stemming from the Yang Long Form

The background on all the various Yang forms is the same, no matter what the conceptual tweaks. They stem from a Yang Long Form that was, well, pretty long for most folks. This form had anywhere from 88 to 108 movements, depending on how you counted them, not to mention all the pieces of each singular movement. Oh, by the way, the 88-movement series was considered simplified. Yeah, uh-huh, 88 is simple? Well, okay, maybe simp*ler* is the real way to put it. Performed properly, these forms could take from 20 to 30 minutes to get through. That's not a lot of time in the grander scheme of things, but first you had to learn this winding, turning, balancing set of moves, which could take years — if you ever really got it down.

T'ai Chi isn't only about memorizing a few steps but also about performing it correctly, with all the right flowing transitions and continuation of chi. Early T'ai Chi devotees were able to dedicate entire lifetimes to learning and perfecting their art because they often started very young and practiced hours a day, sometimes after dealing with life's other demands. But I don't presume that you've bought this book so you can dedicate your life to it. Contemporary life has a lot of other demands, leaving you with maybe a few hours a week for this kind of thing — if you're lucky.

You can use this traditional Yang Short Form as a launch pad to additional T'ai Chi study or other Chinese mind-body arts, such as Qigong. (Find out about Qigong in Chapters 5, 13, and 14.) You can also practice it as an entirely legitimate form all in itself, and it'll keep you very satisfied your entire T'ai Chi life.

Some devout and traditional T'ai Chi students and teachers say that practicing the long form imparts greater health benefits than even several repetitions of a shorter form. But don't discount what you'll gain from a short form practice. Even for the advanced T'ai Chi practitioner, the short form provides a compact "T'ai Chi break" that can be performed in just a few minutes.

And don't be fooled into thinking that, because this is "only the short form," you don't have to pay it as much attention or offer it as much respect. You'll indeed need the same sincere effort as you'd need with any of the longer T'ai Chi forms. So heads up and eyes open throughout.

With fewer moves to learn, you can make every single one count.

A little bit of something is better than a whole lot of nothing. That's how Manny, my collaborator, likes to put it.

Everything long is short again

With the increasing demands of everyday life in China, the culture of T'ai Chi was disappearing from the modern-day masses because of the intimidation of learning such a long, time-consuming set of movements. Fewer and fewer people were practicing T'ai Chi, and as a result, the benefits of physical and mental health were getting lost. Or, maybe I should say, not being found. (See Chapter 2 if you want to find out about the physical and mental benefits.) Noting this dilemma, the Chinese government stepped in. In 1956, China's National Physical Culture and Sports Commission devised a shorter form consisting of 24 movements. Think of it as China's version of T'ai Chi CliffsNotes. The movements were all taken from the traditional Yang Long Form, and they had the feel and applied the same principles of T'ai Chi practice. Nevertheless, these movement were now shorter and more accessible because they took less time to learn — and only about 4–6 minutes or so to move through — and therefore helped preserve a piece of China's heritage.

Taking on the First Part, Yang-Style Short Form

Even 24 smoothly connected moves (which actually each consist of several movements) can be a little mind-boggling, so I divided the entire form into three chapters. This chapter describes the first eight forms.

I know the names sound weird now, but you'll understand better — and they'll roll off your tongue easier — when you move through them and see how they flow together and feel.

Each of these combine the best aspects of the principle of opposites called *yin and yang* — one part of the body retreats while another advances and one part sinks while another rises (see Chapter 7). Each combines attacking-type *(offensive)* movement with defending-type *(defensive)* movement. Put them together and you get a great variety of movement challenges in a few short moments.

Repulse the Monkey (later in this chapter) is a great benefit to anyone with balance problems or to someone who is older. It teaches you to move backwards gracefully and smoothly, something that many people lose with age, after a few sports injuries, or just from simple disuse. So parry that primate for a great connection to your chi and roots.

Each movement flows from one to the next — without stopping. At least that's the theory after you learn each movement. Each move begins from the position and the direction in which the preceding move finishes.

The basic positions and postures that are the foundation to these forms are discussed in depth in Chapter 8. Refer to that chapter for detailed instruction on T'ai Chi Posture, T'ai Chi Hands and Arms, Bow Stance, Centering Step, Empty Step, and Hold Balloon.

Commencement (#1)

Also called Open the Door, or Beginning, or Opening

All the forms, no matter what school or style, start with an opening move that is pretty similar. No, I'm not talking about a handshake, although I suppose you can call this movement a handshake with your chi. The other schools' variations likely differ only in knee bending, timing, or stepping.

Basically, the Commencement helps you gather your energy, find your focus, and breathe fully before beginning the series of movements that make up the form. Whatever its name, use it as shown in Figure 9-1 to bring your mind to the right place for the practice you're about to begin.

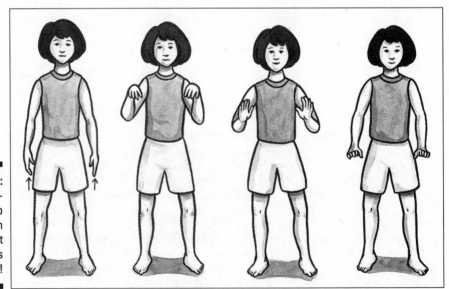

Figure 9-1: Commencement: A cap and gown aren't always involved!

1. **Facing 12 o'clock, start in a narrow stance with your feet together, knees relaxed, and arms loose at your sides.**

   Take this moment to find your tall T'ai Chi Posture and yet relax in all the right spots.

2. **Inhale fully while lifting your arms, moving from the shoulder as your hands move to about shoulder-height (already practicing T'ai Chi hands, of course). At the same time, shift your weight slightly and subtly to the left foot. Keep your elbows soft and rounded.**

3. **As soon as the hands reach the top of the move, exhale and step out with your right foot so your feet are about hip-width apart.**

4. **Sink down slightly with your knees and your entire body weight while exhaling fully. At the same time, let your arms drop slowly and finish at about navel-height, wrists cocked slightly so your palms are facing down.**

   Elbows are still relaxed and softly rounded. Feel the connection to the ground — and to Earth's chi — with the soles of your feet.

   You can repeat this step several times before you begin, if you need a little more time to breathe fully to help you find your focus.

What to avoid:

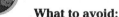

✔ Sticking out your buttocks

✔ Jutting forward with your chin

✔ Standing in a military-like posture with chest puffed outward

✔ Slouching

Parting the Wild Horse's Mane (#2)

Also called Parting the Horse's Mane

As the form's first "real" movement, this one does the job quickly in illustrating the principle of opposites called *yin and yang* that I discuss in Chapters 3 and 7: One arm pushes forward as the other pulls back, and the front arm rises as the body sinks. That's what makes this one form, as shown in Figure 9-2, a wonderful practice or workout all by its lonesome. You can do this form repeatedly by alternating sides while doing it in place or while moving across the room.

The following short form is done three times, starting on the left, moving to the right, and then finishing on the left.

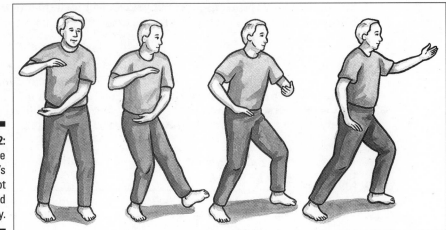

Figure 9-2:
Parting the
Wild Horse's
Mane: Not
so wild
really.

1. **Start facing 12 o'clock, the same way you finished the Commencement.**

2. **Inhale as you shift your weight subtly to the right foot, keeping your knees softly bent.**

3. **Pull your left foot into a Centering Step (see Chapter 8) with the ball of the foot barely grazing the ground next to the right ankle. At the same time, bring your arms into a Hold Balloon position with the right arm, palm down, at chest level and the left arm, palm up, at hip level, arms rounded, ready to hold the balloon between them.**

4. **Exhale as you step out into a Bow Stance with your left foot moving toward 8 o'clock. At the same time, sweep outward and upward diagonally with your left hand and push palm down with your right hand moving to the inside of your left hand.**

   Your palms cross past each other as they move in opposite directions. Your right palm ends facing down at your right hip.

   The left-arm sweep feels a little like you are skipping rocks. The left arm reaches out and up more than the arm rotation of Ward Off in Grasp the Bird's Tail, which is the eighth move of the form as well as the last move in this chapter.

5. **Finish both the forward-stepping and weight-shifting into the Bow Stance to face a 9 o'clock position at the *same* time that your left hand reaches the upward position.**

   Let your eyes follow the forward fingers. The fingers are curved upward slightly, and the palm is facing the front of your heart. Your elbows are still softly rounded.

Breathe out fully each time you shift your weight forward into the Bow Stance with the arm sweep, and breathe in as you shift backward. This helps unblock your chi and relax your muscles.

Now you're ready to repeat this step two more times, moving to your right side and then finishing on your left again, all the while rotating yourself on your personal clock face (see Chapter 8).

6. **Inhale and rock backward, shifting your weight onto your right foot, bending the right knee, and lifting the left toe off the ground. Pivot the left heel to turn the left foot outward so the toe is facing approximately 7 o'clock.**

7. **Drop the toes back to the ground. Then shift your weight back onto the forward foot to make a Centering Step with your weight on your left foot and the right toe grazing the floor next to your left ankle.**

8. **At the same time you are moving into the Centering Step facing 7 o'clock, return your arms to a Hold Balloon position, but this time with the left arm curved gently on top.**

The hands should arrive at the position just as your feet get to their position. But, of course, you just keep flowing through those positions into the next!

9. **Get ready to step out into a Bow Stance again, this time on the opposite side: Exhale as you step out into the stance with your right foot moving toward 10 o'clock. At the same time, sweep outward and upward diagonally with your right hand and push palm down with your left hand moving to the inside of your right hand.**

Your palms cross each other as they move in opposite directions. Your left palm ends facing down at your left hip.

10. **Repeat the entire rock-back sequence to get into the last rock-forward of the Bow Stance: Inhale and rock backward, shifting your weight onto your left foot, bending the left knee, and lifting the right toe off the ground. Pivot the right heel to be able to turn the right foot outward so the toe is facing approximately 11 o'clock.**

11. **Drop the toes back to the ground. Shift your weight back to the forward foot to make a Centering Step with your weight on your right foot and the left toe grazing the floor next to your right ankle.**

12. **At the same time that you are moving into the Centering Step facing about 11 o'clock (near your original position), return your arms to a Hold Balloon position, but this time with the right arm curved gently on top.**

Remember the curve of the elbow. Get ready to step out into your last Wild Horse Bow Stance.

13. **Exhale as you step out into the stance with your left foot moving toward 9 o'clock, just as you did the first time. At the same time, sweep outward and upward diagonally with your left hand and push your palm down with your right hand moving to the inside of your left hand.**

Your palms cross past each other as they move in opposite directions. Your right palm ends facing down at your right hip.

Think this sounds too easy? Then try making the lunge lower with knees more deeply bent. A few minutes of these on either side and you may find yourself mentally challenged to stay focused, as well as physically challenged as your muscles in your legs and torso tire as you ask them to stay low.

What to avoid:

✔ Letting your elbows lock out in an extended position

✔ Forgetting to breathe fully as you rock forward and backward

✔ Allowing your arms to arrive at a position before or after your feet get there

White Crane Cools Its Wings (#3)

Also called Stork Spreading Its Wings or White Crane Spreads Wings

You may think you look like a big bird while you do this movement. There you are, perched on one leg with your wings — er, arms — spread out in different directions. Your right hand is up protecting your head (thanks to T'ai Chi's defensive purpose), and your left hand is down protecting your left hip and side.

This movement, shown in Figure 9-3, can also be practiced as a stationary stance on both sides; hold it for several breath cycles and then change sides. This helps train for better balance.

This step also incorporates a little twist with the waist without the feet moving as you move the arms. It can be tricky to coordinate, but a bit of practice does wonders for your program!

1. **Start from the last position of the previous form; in this case, the Parting-Mane Bow Stance facing approximately 9 o'clock, with left arm forward and right arm down at hip.**

With your lower body, you do a slick little weight change to go from the Bow Stance to an Empty Step. I call it the Bow-To-Empty Transition. That's not an official name, by the way, but because this transition comes up several times, I present it separately in Chapter 8 as one of the transitions.

When you twist slightly through your waist from to the right and then to the left at the end of the transition, move your arms into a Hold Balloon position with your left arm on top. But don't keep your arms holding that little balloon! Keep them flowing to the next position.

Flowing through the Hold Balloon means that if you were observing, you may not notice this form unless you knew that Hold Balloon was there.

2. **Let the right hand move upward on a vertical line grazing just past the outside of the left hand's little finger.**

The hand stops at forehead height with palm facing in (because you're protecting yourself).

I learned from Manny that the movement of the right arm feels like doing an inside block in defensive martial arts. If you aren't familiar with that stuff, just imagine someone coming at you and then react by raising your arm to keep him or her from hitting you. You can also imagine your right palm as a mirror that you are looking into to check your hairdo.

3. **While the right hand is going up, the left hand moves downward on a vertical line to hip-height, palm facing down.**

At the same time your hands move apart from the Hold Balloon position, you rock back fully onto your right foot to create the Empty Step. Body and eyes face 9 o'clock.

What to avoid:

- ✔ Hurrying into the Empty Step
- ✔ Letting the hands move outward, not just up and down
- ✔ Leaning back with the upper body on the first subtle step-in weight-shift

Brush Knees (#4)

Also called Brushing Your Knees and Stepping or Brush Knee and Push

Without fancy horses' manes to part or lutes playing games with you, this movement sounds simple. Brushing knees takes its name from the front hand passing down the front leg and brushing in front of the knee, like a low blocking technique in a defensive Chinese martial art. But the emphasis is on the rear hand pushing, or striking, forward. Your body sinks below the push to unleash more power.

This movement is a good illustration of a Taoist aphorism: "All streams flow to the sea because it is lower than they are. Humility gives it its power."

Sink as you Brush Knees so your power can rise, rise, rise. Refer to Figure 9-4 to see how much you can rise.

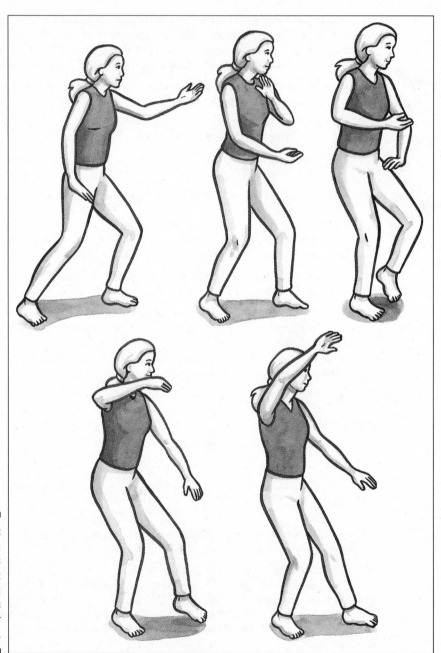

Figure 9-3:
White Crane
Cools Its
Wings:
Waving
your arms
around for
better chi.

Don't be daunted by the length of this movement! Brush Knees is the same movement repeated three times, alternating sides. I try to make it easier by breaking it apart: First focus on just the right arm and then just the left arm. Then add the footwork, which (surprise!) is exactly the same as the alternating footwork of the Bow Stances in Parting the Horse's Mane.

1. **Start from the final posture of White Crane, facing 9 o'clock.**

   You move both arms at the same time, but I describe one and then the other to clarify.

2. **First, the right arm: Circle the right arm downward, rotating the arm completely from the shoulder joint so the elbow stays softly rounded. The palm faces up and your waist rotates to the right as the arm moves downward.**

   Keep the circling going, palm rotating to stay facing upward, as the arm continues the circle back up until it is extended outward at shoulder-height. The front of your body faces 11 o'clock, and your hand is outreached at about 1 o'clock with eyes also in that direction.

3. **The left arm now has to be coordinated with the right arm: At the same time that the right arm is circling downward and then upward to 1 o'clock, rotate the left forearm from the elbow joint so the hand drops downward then circles around and back to the left and up to about nose-height. It then drops back down to the right to chest-height with palm down. Your left elbow is also lifted to chest-height.**

   Relax through the back and spine so you can twist ever so slightly to the right and left through the waist with your arms. Bending your knees helps.

4. **Now's the time to start rotating around yourself using the Bow Stances: Step outward and forward with your left foot to 8 o'clock to make the first of three Bow Stances. At the same time, leave the right elbow high and bend at the elbow to push with the palm past your cheek and out to the front of you at eye level.**

   Imagine that you are pushing away an opponent.

5. **At the same time (don't you get tired of that piece of instruction?), your left arm continues its circling downward across your chest, and down toward your knee (there's the Brush Knee part!). The left hand finishes, palm facing down, at hip-height.**

6. **To move into the second of the series of three Brush Knee steps, rock your weight backward onto your right foot, letting the right knee bend — now the feet completely mimic Horse's Mane — and lift your left toes, rotate the left foot outward to about 7 o'clock by pivoting on the left heel, and return the toes to the ground.**

7. **Shift your weight back to the forward foot to make a Centering Step with your weight on your left foot and the right toe grazing the floor next to your left ankle.**

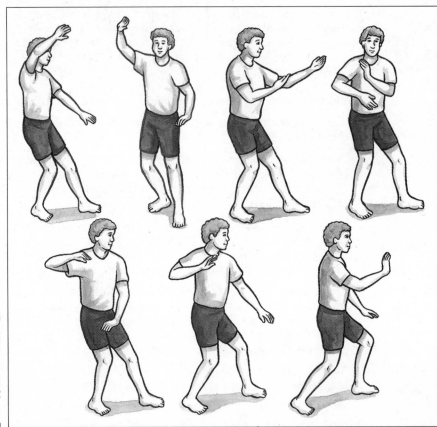

Figure 9-4:
Brush
Knees: You
kneed to
brush past
your knees.

8. **At the same time that you are moving into the Centering Step facing 7 o'clock, your arms rotate just as they earlier in this form.**

   Your arms do the same movements, but they switch sides: The left one does what the right one did (circling down and reaching to the back with elbow high and palm up), and the right one does what the left one did (circling down and back up to chest-height, also with elbow high, but with the palm down).

   Think of these as three separate steps. Then link them mentally and physically to help you through the progression.

9. **Now you get to move into your second Bow Stance: Step forward to 10 o'clock with your right foot. At the same time, leave the right elbow high and bend at the elbow to push with the palm past your cheek and out to the front of you at eye level. Your left arm continues its circling downward across your chest, and down toward your knee to finish with palm facing down at hip-height.**

Here comes the heel pivot and Centering Step transition to move into your last Bow Stance with Brush Knee:

10. **Rock your weight backward onto your left foot letting the left knee bend. Lift your right toes, rotate the right foot outward to 11 o'clock (back to your front) by pivoting on the right heel, and then return the toes to the ground.**

    With all the rocking back and forth, this is a great form to practicing inhaling on the rock back and exhaling on the rock forward.

11. **Shift your weight back to the forward foot to make a Centering Step facing about 12 o'clock with your weight on your right foot and the left toe grazing the floor next to your right ankle.**

12. **At the same time you are moving into the Centering Step, your arms rotate just as they did the first time through (see Steps 2 and 3).**

13. **Finish by stepping outward and forward with your left foot to 8 o'clock to make the first of three Bow Stances. At the same time, leave the right elbow high and bend at the elbow to push with the palm past your cheek and out to the front of you at eye level.**

What to avoid:

- ✔ Locking the elbow when you brush with the palm forward
- ✔ Thinking too hard about the arms (because the circling motion moves naturally)
- ✔ Not breathing with the rocking and weight-shifting forward and backward

Strum the Lute (#5)

Also called Playing the Pi'pa or Play the Guitar

This is a deceptively simple move during which you get to try the Empty Step (refer to Chapter 8). Imagining that you are holding a stringed instrument between your hands can help you visualize the proper hand placement, as shown in Figure 9-5.

Strumming and lifting

When Strum the Lute is performed with the right hand and right foot forward, it's called Lifting Hands. You see, the old masters gave these movements names that would be more easily remembered than would a lengthy description of the technique. So such names as "Strum the Lute" and "Lifting Hands" became verbal shorthand for the same techniques performed on opposite sides. That's another little story from Manny, my collaborator.

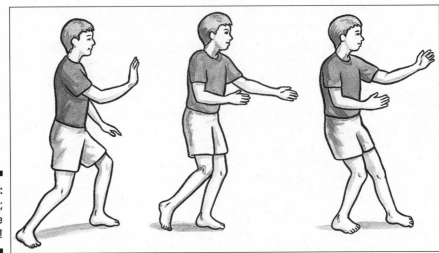

Figure 9-5:
Give a hoot;
Strum the
Lute!

It was said of the old T'ai Chi masters that their movements were not fancy, but their strikes were like a mountain falling. That's because of the power that can be achieved by perfect balance and placement, not just brute force.

Lute-strumming — or Pi'pa playing, if you prefer — is another posture that can be practiced as a stationary stance. It is a good movement to develop the flow of your chi. When you do it in isolation rather than as a part of the entire 24 forms, hold the position with the left hand and left foot forward for five inhales and exhales and then switch sides and do the same. Strum the Lute just 10 minutes each day, and you'll eventually accumulate chi force in your hands. Let the Force be with you!

1. **Start facing 9 o'clock in the final position of Brush Knee. Step forward with your right foot about a half-foot length while you slowly (what else is new?) bring your left hand forward, moving it from the shoulder and rotating the palm from facing down to facing in or across your body.**

2. **Rock your weight onto your right leg as you bend that knee, letting your upper body rotate naturally to the right to about 10 o'clock. At the same time, lift your left foot and then return just the toe to lightly graze the ground without any weight on it.**

   You have created an Empty Step. This transition is much like the Bow-to-Empty transition that I describe in Chapter 8.

3. **At the same time your feet are moving, your arms are moving toward their positions with the upper body turning back toward your legs: The left arm continues its movement until it is extended about shoulder-height with the palm facing in and the elbow nearly extended but still curved.**

You should feel as if you were about to shake hands with somebody, but with the left arm.

4. **Your right arm pulls backward with the elbow pulling down slightly. The right palm also faces in and finishes just below and to your right of your left elbow. You finish facing 9 o'clock.**

A tall but relaxed posture with your tailbone pulled down can help you stay balanced and not sway.

What to avoid:

- Putting weight on your front left foot
- Straightening your right knee

Repulse the Monkey (#6)

Also called Fending off the Monkey or Step Back, Repulse Monkey

As if a monkey is in your living room? People like this step — although it's one of the hardest — because of the odd name. Believe me, I really didn't make up these names! As shown in Figure 9-6, this is an essential exercise for developing the skill to move backwards gracefully and balanced — a skill that is lost due to aging or lack of practice.

1. **Start in the final position of Strum the Lute in which your weight is on your right foot to the rear and your hands are forward as if holding the stringed instrument. Your entire body still faces 9 o'clock.**

2. **Turn your right hand palm up and circle it downward and to the rear in a large arc that moves all the way behind you to 2 o'clock. Turn your waist toward 12 o'clock with the arm circle, as your eyes follow the hand.**

3. **When your hand reaches about shoulder-height to the rear, bring the palm straight in to brush past your cheek as if you are pushing something away to your front. Your elbow should bend at an acute angle when the hand brushes past your ear. Your waist rotates back toward 9 o'clock with the rear-circling arm movement.**

Your palm is cupped and sort of grazes near your ear on its path forward as if you are trying to hear something better.

4. **At the moment your right hand moves past your ear, step back with your left foot, touching your toes first, and then rolling back onto the entire foot with your weight, to create another Empty Step with your right foot forward. Realign your new front foot so your toes face forward.**

5. **Your right hand continues to float forward, turning palm down as your left hand now turns palm up.**

The two palms float past each other, with your right one continuing its path forward, and your left one now starting its journey to the rear to repeat the entire process starting with Step 2 on the opposite side.

6. **Repeat the step four times — right, left, and then again right, left, traveling backward with each step.**

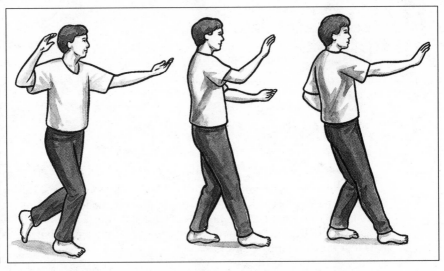

Figure 9-6:
Repulse the Monkey: No, it doesn't mean that the orangutan won't like you.

What to avoid:

✔ Letting your backward-stepping and hand-cupping sweep be disconnected.

✔ Clunking down with your step backward instead of quietly and softly placing your foot on the floor.

✔ Moving your foot as you step backward across your body's midline.

Grasp the Bird's Tail — Left (#7)

Also called Grasping the Sparrow's Tail

This simple-sounding form, beautifully enough, covers half the key movements of T'ai Chi and has four parts — Ward Off, Roll Back, Press, and Push — some of which have several parts themselves. Be sure to practice this form on both sides. You can spend entire sessions doing this one move on both sides over and over! Figure 9-7 shows you all the parts for both the left side and the right side, which is the next set of instruction.

THERESE'S TWO CENTS

Doubly repulsing

Manny, my intrepid collaborator, says that his teacher instructed his class to do Repulse the Monkey from one end of the park to the other and then turn around and "repulse" all the way back again. Yeah, you may feel a little funny doing that in public, and no, you can't do it without attracting attention. But you can gain all kinds of balance and grace goodies with that kind of repetition.

Note that this move has names for its four parts (I put the names in the instruction so you know where they are). The names are: Ward Off, Roll Back, Press, and Push. Use them as great devices for the progression of steps, because they aptly describe what you do in each segment.

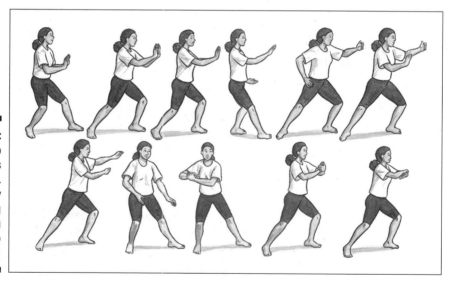

Figure 9-7:
Grasp
the Bird's
Tail — Left.
As if any
bird is going
to let you
hang onto
its tail!

1. **Rotate your body from the closing position (facing 9 o'clock) of Repulse the Monkey to return to face your front to 12 o'clock. Inhale during the rotation. Keep your weight on your right foot so you can draw your left foot in to a Centering Step.**

2. **At the same time, draw in your arms to a Hold Balloon position with right arm on top, palm down, and left arm at hip-height, palm facing up.**

3. **Exhale and step out into a Bow Stance, as in the first form, with the left foot leading out toward 8 o'clock.**

4. **Ward Off: At the same time you step out into the Bow Stance, extend your left hand in front of you with the palm cupped and facing you at chest-height. Point your thumb upward so your elbow is dropped slightly.**

   Your right hand is palm down at your right hip with the elbow bent slightly. (This is where the Bird's Tail gets grasped, so to speak.)

   The hands may seem similar to the first part of Wild Horse's Mane at first (see the section, "Parting The Wild Horse's Mane," which is the first move after the opening), but pay close attention, and you'll feel and see the difference. You can also check out Figure 9-7, which illustrates the differences.

5. **Roll Back: Turn your left palm down and your right palm up simultaneously as you reach forward with your right hand until both palms are on the same plane (8 o'clock direction still) at about chest-height. Your right palm is near your left elbow.**

6. **Turn your waist to the right as if you are trying to shine a headlight in the middle of your chest toward about 2 o'clock. At the same time, shift your weight to your right leg, dropping both hands in a low arc in front of you, ending with both hands also facing 2 o'clock, right palm still up and left palm still down.**

7. **Press: Rotate back to the left from your waist. At the same time, round your left arm as it moves outward to 8 o'clock, palm in, and press with your right hand toward your left wrist, barely grazing it.**

8. **Now shift your weight to your left leg until you return to the Bow Stance and press your hands forward.**

   Avoid letting your knee extend beyond your toes when you lunge forward in the Bow Stance, because this can put stress on the tendons of the knee. Your knee should stay behind your toes whenever you bend, and your lower leg should be straight up and down from the ground.

9. **Push: Rotate your hands so you can slide your right palm over the top of your left wrist. (Some teachers reach to forearm.) Then, as you shift your weight to your right leg again, separate the hands to about shoulder-width at navel-height, palms facing down. When your weight is on your back foot, you lift your left toe from the floor.**

10. **Now rock your weight forward onto your left leg again and, at the same time, raise your palms to where they are facing away from you.**

    You should look as if you're preparing to push a really heavy tall object away from you. Your elbows do not actually flex or extend. The arm movement comes from the shoulders.

    On the pushing part, let your body weight sink into the ground, letting your power rise from the back heel as you bring more chi energy into your body.

11. Transition to the right side by using the Sweep Open transition that I describe in Chapter 8: Shift your weight onto your right foot, keeping the knee bent, and turn to the right. Open your body fully to face 12 o'clock. At the same time, float both arms open and out to each side, palms facing out, as if you are a bird trying a single flap of the wings. Your left foot rotates in so the left toes also face 12 o'clock.

12. Shift your weight back to your left foot and draw your right toes in to a Centering Step. At the same time, bring your arms to a Hold Balloon position with left arm on top.

What to avoid:

🖊 Allowing your elbows to straighten or lock

🖊 Jerking or halting between each of the movements without coordinating all the turning, lifting, and weight-shifting.

Grasp the Bird's Tail — Right (#8)

This form is exactly the same as the preceding tail-grasping form, but on the opposite side. Coordinating both arms and feet is complex, so I translate the sides for you so you don't have to try to switch the instructions in your head.

1. Start from the closing position of the transition on the left side in the preceding set of instructions.

2. Exhale and step out into a Bow Stance, as in the first form, with the right foot leading out toward 4 o'clock.

3. Ward Off: At the same time you step out into the Bow Stance, extend your right hand in front of you with the palm cupped and facing you at chest-height. Point your thumb upward so your elbow is dropped slightly. Your left hand is palm down at your left hip with the elbow bent slightly.

4. Roll Back: Turn your right palm down and your left palm up simultaneously as you reach forward with your left hand until both palms are on the same plane (4 o'clock direction still) at about chest-height. Your left palm is near your right elbow.

If you start to feel your back tighten up in any way on this part of the move, bend both knees a little more so you free up more motion in your spine.

5. Turn your waist to the left so your chest faces about 2 o'clock. At the same time, shift your weight to your left leg, dropping both hands in a low arc in front of you, ending with both hands also facing 2 o'clock, left palm still up and right palm still down.

6. **Press:** Rotate back to the right from your waist. At the same time, round your right arm as it moves outward to 4 o'clock, palm in, and press with your left hand toward your right wrist.

7. Shift your weight to your right leg until you return to the Bow Stance and press your hands forward.

8. **Push:** Rotate your hands so you can slide your left palm over the top of your right wrist. Then, as you shift your weight to your left leg again, separate the hands to about shoulder-width at navel-height, palms facing down. When your weight is on your back foot, lift your right toe from the floor.

9. Rock your weight forward onto your right leg again, and at the same time, raise your palms to where they are facing away from you as if preparing to push something away.

Your elbows do not actually flex or extend. The arm movement comes from the shoulders.

When doing all the forms, if you don't think so hard and just let your body move naturally, you flow through them much easier.

In Chapter 10, I show you the next seven moves of the Yang Short Form. As always, the next movement leads off from the position in which this one ends.

Chapter 10

Keeping the Flow, Yang-Style

. . . .

In This Chapter

▶ Thinking about your style of learning

▶ Taking on the second part of the Yang Short Form

▶ Learning how to drop your hand, T'ai Chi-style

. . . .

*W*ith the first eight movements of the form under your belt, you're ready to move on. Okay, okay, I know that you don't have all the movements down cold — yet. Really, that's just fine. You're just terribly eager to see what comes next, right?

In Chapter 8, I review the basic stuff, such as what to do with your feet and hands so you don't get all tangled up and fall down in a heap. In Chapter 9, I discuss the first eight forms of this 24-form style, including some key movements, such as Grasp the Bird's Tail and Parting the Wild Horse's Mane (moves that demonstrate many of the principles of T'ai Chi). In this chapter, I move on to the next seven forms.

> Single Whip
>
> Wave Hands Like Clouds
>
> Single Whip
>
> Pat the High Horse
>
> Kick with Right Heel
>
> Strike Opponents Ears with Both Fists
>
> Kick with Left Heel

From some of those seven forms comes a couple of favorites:

> ✔ **Kicks with Heels:** My personal choice, these kicks feel so powerful and help me feel so grounded no matter how low or high the leg goes. While in motion, I like the challenge of lifting my leg — in slow motion, no less, — but staying rooted and balanced. Well, I can do it sometimes. Oh, and you get to do this twice.

> ✔ **Wave Hands Like Clouds:** Manny's personal pick — I think that he just picked this one because of the heavenly name. He says that this movement is just dandy as a workout all by itself, repeated over and over, or even as a warm-up. He also says that he sometimes does it first thing in the morning, moving from one end of the room to the other and then back, waving his hands like clouds the entire time. I haven't seen my collaborator at his morning hand-waving, so I'll just have to take his word for it.

Determining How You Want to Learn

Learning T'ai Chi — and other Chinese mind-body arts like Qigong can be very foreign to the minds and bodies of most Westerners. In the first class I took, the teacher never really explained anything. He just said, "Okay, let's go," so we all followed him the best we could. He sort of assumed that we knew what he meant.

But I had so many questions: What does this mean? Why am I doing it? Why are you saying face north when we aren't? A couple times, I tried to ask a question, but he didn't seem to understand why I'd need to ask. So I just learned to go with it, following the flow and trying to ignore the questions swimming in my head.

My first experience is a pretty accurate example of the differences between learning a mind-body art the Chinese way and learning one the Western way. Chinese (remember, I'm generalizing!) just accept it and flow with it, moving through a form while also giving full attention to the inner details of chi, energy flow, and principles of T'ai Chi movement. Westerners, however, want to break down each form, question the movement of each little finger, and learn the mechanics before turning much attention to flow or mindfulness.

There are a lot of very complicated approaches to learning styles. Heck, you can spend an entire college degree studying them! Take the time now to think about how you want to learn T'ai Chi or about which learning style is best for your personality. You can even take a moment to think about how'd you feel in a situation with the opposite style!

> ✔ Learning the Chinese way may take a long, long time because trying to feel the energy itself can take months, years, or much of a lifetime. So learning a T'ai Chi sequence properly and performing it correctly can take a lifetime. A lifetime? Oh my!

> ✔ Learning the Western way — for Westerners at least — can give you a quicker feeling of satisfaction and of having accomplished something. In this case, the accomplishment is the mechanical movement. You work your way through the external movement and limb placement and then go back and try to add your chi and all the T'ai Chi principles.

Manny finds that his students (mostly Westerners) prefer the second method, so he obliges them by breaking it all down. He'd rather not, but it seems to keep students coming back long enough to begin to understand. And they still get the mindful and healthful benefits no matter how they set about learning T'ai Chi.

Manny has had students who — like me — wanted to question every little muscle twitch with a resounding "Why?" Sometimes, he tells them just to do the forms without constant questions or analysis and then come tell *him* the "why" in a couple of weeks. Works like a charm — "Sometimes," Manny says, "you just have to get the left brain out of the way."

There are no shortcuts in T'ai Chi or even in Qigong. You need to cultivate your chi and its flow to fully realize all the benefits.

With that in mind, think about your best style of learning as you take on the next part of the Yang 24-Movement Short Form.

Learning the Second Part, Yang-Style Short Form

This chapter contains forms 9 through 15. Two of them repeat as separate forms, so this section isn't as long to work through. Nevertheless, take the time to move through each one thoroughly, trying to truly feel the flow and balance and beginning to let your body recognize the movement patterns — without thinking too hard.

Don't miss the favorites! Kick with Heel and Wave Hands Like Clouds.

The basic movements, stances, and positions for feet, hands, arms, and posture are in Chapter 8. So refer to that chapter whenever you need to refresh your memory about a basic form.

Single Whip (#9)

Also called Simple Whip

Call this T'ai Chi's signature stance because, to most people who don't know anything about T'ai Chi, the Single Whip looks like what they imagine T'ai Chi to look like. But it's not easy, because both hands are held differently, which really taxes the brain to manage them both — sort of like rubbing your stomach and patting your head. Take the time to learn the Single Whip: It's not only a great way to feel grounded but it also forces full and controlled breathing.

The next time someone asks you to "Show me some T'ai Chi," you can proudly step through this movement and impress them a little, too.

Figure 10-1 helps you get the hang of the Single Whip. Feel the power of sinking into the back foot so you're like a loaded spring.

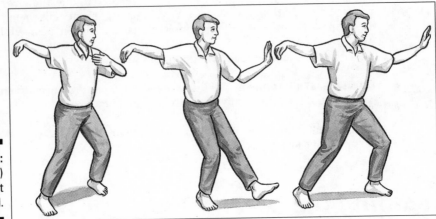

Figure 10-1:
(Single)
Whip it
good.

1. **Start in the concluding position for Grasp the Bird's Tail — Right (see Chapter 9) with right foot forward facing 3 or 4 o'clock and right palms forward in the Push position.**

2. **Let your weight shift to your left foot while turning your body through the waist to face about 11 o'clock. While the body is turning, lift the right toes and pivot the foot on its heel so the toes turn to face about 11 o'clock also. At the same time, turn your right palm to face you and let the left hand float downward in an arc, all moving with the pivot of the right foot.**

   Be sure to lift the toes for the foot-pivot so you don't torque your knee in ways it shouldn't be moved and won't much like.

3. **Begin moving your arms into a Hold Balloon position with the right arm on top and then start shifting your weight back onto your right foot, sinking into the bent knee. Finish by pulling in the left toe to a Centering Step.**

4. **Float the left hand, palm in, in front of the face at about nose-height (and think of the opponent you are blocking), while you move the right hand to your side (about 2 o'clock) and relax the wrist into a Dropped Hand position with fingers together (see Figure 8-6 in Chapter 8). The elbow is also bent and dropped downward slightly.**

You never want to have your hands right in front of your eyes so you can't see your opponent. (Remember, even if you aren't kicking teeth, you have to imagine the moves as if you are, because T'ai Chi stems from defensive needs and training. Check out Chapter 1 for more information.) They should be just below your eyes in most cases, so you can peek over the top while still protecting yourself, so to speak.

5. **Lift your left toe and step outward to about 8 o'clock into a Bow Stance while your left hand sweeps out to your side also, palm out, to about 9 o'clock.**

Think of the body-crossing sweep with your left hand as another blocking and striking maneuver. That should help you better visualize the step. Some teachers will indeed ask students to push with the left hand. Keep that in mind as you learn. Nobody's wrong, just different. You have to determine what you like best. (See Chapter 4 for more information about different schools and styles.)

What to avoid:

✔ Stiffening through the shoulders or elbows, especially with the Dropped Hand

✔ Lifting the Dropped Hand higher or dropping it lower than about shoulder-height

Wave Hands Like Clouds (#10)

Also called Move Hands Like Clouds

If time is short or if you can't manage enough energy (or memory) to do the form, do a series of Wave Hands Like Clouds (refer to Figure 10-2) for whatever time you do have — even as a mini-stress break during the day. Find an isolated stairwell or a back hallway and just starting waving.

This is Manny's favorite form. Maybe because while practicing this form — after doing T'ai Chi for more than a year — he got in touch with his chi. He says his hands suddenly "felt full," which means that he was manifesting his chi through his *acupoints,* which I like to call to call your body's energy superhighway on- and off-ramps (for more detail, check out Chapter 13). Maybe you'll have the same experience after you've been waving awhile.

One thing that may help you have a chi-manifesting experience is to breathe fully. Breathing fully means that you make sure your breath goes deep into your lungs and inflates your abdomen, rather than just a little shallow puff-puff into your chest. For more on breathing, visit Chapters 3, 4 and 13. In this form, you want to exhale as you shift your weight to the left, and inhale as you close with your right foot.

Dropping the Hand

This name describes the hallmark hand position that seems to scream T'ai Chi! It's not just dropping the hand, however, or "hooking" it, as you may also hear it called. This movement is the entire interplay between wrist, hand, and fingers. Frankly, it reminds me of a duck's beak. Try doing a Donald Duck shadow play on the walls, with your fingers being the top of the beak and your thumb being the bottom. Now just drop the fingers from your wrist so they face the ground instead of being parallel to the ground, and pull all the fingertips closed (so Donald can't talk).

That's basically what a Dropped Hand looks like. (See Chapter 8 for details on the Dropped Hand position.)

People have different styles, some with straighter fingers, some more curved, and some more "dropped" in the wrist than others. But for now, as a novice, just start to get the feel. It takes enough to get one hand into this position while the other is doing something else, and you're still moving your legs, too.

One little point to keep repeating to yourself: Go left. In other words, steps go left in Wave Hands Like Clouds in sort of a sideways heel-toe shuffle pattern with feet basically parallel. Go left, go left, go left . . .

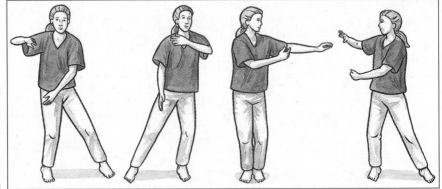

Figure 10-2:
Wave
Hands Like
Clouds: Hi,
mom!

1. **From the last position of Single Whip, shift your weight back to your right foot, letting the knee bend and your body weight sink. At the same time, lift the left toes, pivot on the heel so the toes face forward, and rotate your torso to about 1 o'clock. While the feet are shifting, your left arm floats downward in an arc and back up to your right side to about shoulder level and slightly away from your body. Your right hand (the one in Dropped Hand) opens to a soft T'ai Chi Hand (see Chapter 8).**

Now you're ready to start the smooth hand-waving and side-stepping of Wave Hands.

During this movement, imagine your hands tracing two circles in front of you with the center of the circle at each shoulder joint. The circles are sort of like two hula hoops hanging flat in front of your body with their center at shoulder-height.

2. **Drop your right hand downward so the palm is facing your navel as you shift your weight back to your left foot (exhale), bringing in the right foot to join it (inhale) so they're about a fist width apart.**

   Let your torso move to the front with the side-stepping, and be sure to carry the arms with your torso.

   Check to make sure that you have space between your body and your upper arm, as if you are holding a balloon in place.

3. **Exchange the hand positions so the right one lifts and the left one drops, exactly opposite of the arms in Step 2.**

4. **Rotate from the waist to the right slightly as you subtly shift your weight onto your right foot — but don't move the placement of the feet yet! As your waist rotates, carry the hands with the torso back toward the right.**

   That's one step. You do this three times, keeping the exhale and inhale pattern going, too.

   Bent knees during the side-steps helps you root yourself to the ground and keep you from toppling over or just getting wobbly.

5. **Start the next step by stepping out with the left foot, keeping your weight finely balanced on your right, and again switch the arms: Drop the right hand and lift the left hand.**

6. **Shift your weight back to your left foot, letting the right foot join it, and let your torso move to the front with the side-step with the arms.**

7. **Repeat Step 3 and Step 4 one time apiece before you finish with your feet parallel, right hand lifted, torso turned ever so slightly to the right, and your weight shifted to your right foot. You should be facing about 1 o'clock.**

What to avoid:

- Shifting your weight so suddenly that it throws you off balance
- Holding your breath

Single Whip (#11)

This movement is not so complicated. You just get to repeat the Single Whip you did earlier. (See Figure 10-1 to refresh your memory.) The following instruction helps you transition into Single Whip from Wave Hands Like Clouds.

1. Start in the finishing position of Wave Hands Like Clouds. Be sure to still have your weight on your right foot.

2. Instead of switching hands, move back into the start of Step 4 of the prior Single Whip (Form #9), earlier in this chapter. (Your left hand moves slightly upward and in front of your shoulder, and your right arm, wrist, hand, and fingers go into the Dropped Hand position. Your left toe draws in so you're in another Centering Step.)

3. Lift your left foot and toes to step outward to about 8 o'clock into a Bow Stance. Your left hand sweeps (not pushes) out to your left side — palm out — to about 9 o'clock. Your right hand stays in the Dropped Hand position.

Pat the High Horse (#12)

Also called Patting the Horse's Neck While Riding and High Pat on the Horse

Patting horses looks and feels very much like the previous form in Chapter 9 in which the White Crane Spreads Its Wings. In fact, from the waist down, they are totally identical. So where does the horse come into this? In the placement of the right hand. You reach forward as though you are, well, patting a horse on the side of the neck with your right hand. Nice horsey. Want a carrot?

Now you know what I mean about having a better feeling for these names after you get moving, right? The names are completely literal. Just use your imagination, and you can see the action described. Take a look at Figure 10-3 if you need to see the action on paper for horse-patting.

1. **Start in the finishing position of Single Whip.**

   That's a Bow Stance facing about 8 o'clock, with left hand out in front at 9 o'clock and right hand in the Dropped Hand position behind you at about 2 o'clock.

2. **Here comes another Bow-To-Empty Step transition again (I describe this position in Chapter 8). Here, however, at the same time your right foot begins to move, relax your right hand and turn both right and left palms upward.**

3. **Turn your body at the waist just a bit to the left to kind of square off the Empty Step. At the same time, move your right hand past your ear and to the front. (Pat the horse here!) Your left elbow withdraws back to your side so the left hand is at your left hip, still with its palm up. Your left toe now returns to graze the ground in the Empty Step.**

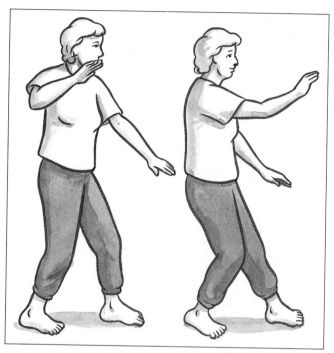

Figure 10-3:
Get off your
high horse
and get this
down pat.

What to avoid:

✔ Putting weight on your left toe in the Empty Step

✔ Rounding your shoulders forward as you pat the horse

Kick with Right Heel (#13)

Also called Separate Hands and Kick, Step Up and Kick, or Heel Kick

Instead of staying well-grounded with both feet on the floor the whole time
(well, almost), you get to kick up your legs — one at a time, of course.
Frankly, this "kick" is less of a kick than you may think, because it's in slow
motion, T'ai Chi style. It's more of a lift of the knee, followed by the lower leg
lifting up, as shown in Figure 10-4. And this movement is a lot harder because
you can't use momentum!

1. **Start in the concluding horse-patting Empty Step position facing 9
   o'clock.**

2. **Rotate your body toward 8 o'clock in a prep movement while you
   bring your arms in to cross your hands at the wrists, left hand with
   palm facing your chest on the inside of the right hand with the palm
   facing out. They are in front of your chest.**

When your right leg is kicking, your left wrist is on the inside (closer to you) or on top. When your left leg is kicking, your right wrist is on the inside (closer to you) or on top. Opposites again (see Chapters 3 and 7 for more details on the principles of yin and yang).

3. **Lift the left toe out of the Empty Step and step forward into a Bow Stance toward 9 o'clock. At the same time, separate your wrists and circle both hands outward and then downward to trace a small circle.**

   The hands finish, both palms up, left wrist on top of right wrist, about 6 inches in front of your navel.

4. **While your arms are finishing their circling downward, bring your right toe to the side of your left ankle in a Centering Step.**

5. **Your right knee now lifts diagonally to about 10 o'clock without shifting your body in any way. Then, keeping your lifted knee firmly stationary in the air, straighten out the lifted lower leg away from you. Think of the right knee as a hinge. Kick or push your heel out (while imagining that your opponent is standing there!) so the foot is flexed.**

6. **At the same time as the leg movement, your arms start to fan upward from the shoulders as the wrists rotate and your palms are facing out (so you can repel an opponent, of course). Then your hands separate, palms out, finishing nose-height at about the 7 o'clock and 10 o'clock corners. Let your eyes follow your right hand. Note that your right arm is at the same outward angle as your right leg.**

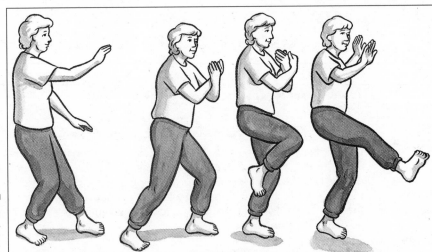

Figure 10-4:
Kick up your
(right) heel.

Lift your kicking leg only as high as you can while still maintaining your spinal alignment. You should be able to almost straighten your lower leg at the knee without slumping, too.

Slumping and tucking your pelvis under weakens you and makes you vulnerable to an opponent, who may just knock you off your feet. No need to be worried about Hollywood-style heels to the nose. Place the pelvis strongly, and it'll do what it needs to do.

What to avoid:

- ✔ Sinking in the ribs or slumping through your back as you kick
- ✔ Locking the knee joint of the standing leg

Strike Opponent's Ears with Both Fists (#14)

Also called Box Both Ears or Hitting Your Opponent with Both Fists

What you get to imagine during this movement is kind of brutal. But here goes: It's as if you are pulling your opponent's head down toward your lifting knee so you can use both fists to strike his or her head, as shown in Figure 10-5. Ouch!

Don't be too appalled. T'ai Chi was — and can still be — used to train people to defend themselves (see Chapter 1). T'ai Chi is, at its roots, a *martial art,* which means hitting and kicking to protect yourself. It so happens that T'ai Chi is often practiced mindfully, as you are here.

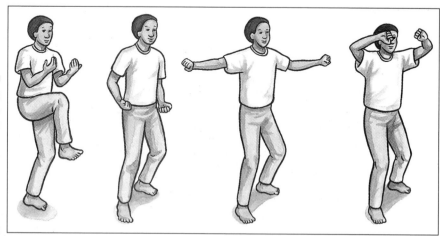

Figure 10-5: Strike Opponent's Ears with Both Fists — then round the bases for a homerun!

1. **Start in the closing position of Kick with Right Heel, facing about 9 o'clock. Your right leg is lifted in the kicking position.**

2. **Bend the right knee so the foot pulls in at a point where the right thigh is parallel with the ground. At the same time, bring both arms**

toward your body, rotating the elbows in so they are close to your side, palms facing up. Your hands end at the same level as your thigh, near your knee.

3. **Still looking straight ahead (you gotta throw off your opponent, you know), inhale and bend the standing left knee and softly bring the right foot toward the ground; then (without actually touching the ground) place the foot on the ground at about 10 o'clock with the right knee straightening as you exhale. Your weight is over your left leg. At the same time, lower your hands (with the palms up) to your side or to about hip-height.**

Keep the flow going on the moves in these steps. They move naturally from one to another without having to tax your brain too much. Now get ready, here comes the power play.

4. **Slowly move both hands into fists as you inhale and shift your weight forward onto the right foot into a Bow Stance toward 10 o'clock. As you shift your weight forward, exhale and lift the arms and fists up and forward so the fists stop at about eye-level in front of your face and have about the width of a head between them. Turn the knuckles in slightly from the wrist.**

What to avoid:

- ✔ Tensing your shoulders and elbows upward in the final position
- ✔ Clenching your fists
- ✔ Rounding your back

Kick with Left Heel (#15)

Also called Separate Hands and Kick, Step Up and Kick, or Heel Kick

Now you get to repeat the kick you did in form #13, but this time on the left side! Gotta stay balanced, you know. Take a look at the reversed figure in Figure 10-6 to help you think through the other side. I provide a description for the other side so it's easier for you to think through, too.

In battle, kicks are used in moderation, which is a lot different from Hollywood's portrayal of flying kicks every which way. Here's another good point about kicks: They may seem powerful, but they can be just the opposite.

- ✔ They leave you potentially off-balance as you stand on one foot.
- ✔ They expose — er, how do I say this? — tender vital areas to the opponent.

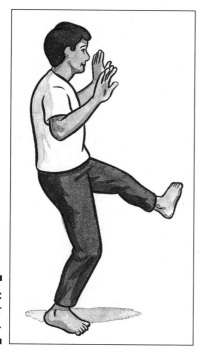

Figure 10-6:
Kick up your
(left) heel.

1. Start in a Bow Stance facing 10 o'clock with arms and fists raised.

2. Transition to where you can do the kick by using the Sweep Open Transition that I describe in Chapter 8: Shift your weight back to your left leg, sinking fully into the left knee. Open your hands so the palms face out and fingers point in toward each other.

3. Rotate your body to the left (sweep open) to about 8 o'clock and pull your hands apart, circling them open and slightly wider as your body turns. Your right toes also turn in.

4. Shift your weight back to your right foot while your arms continue to circle downward. Move your left toe in while you stand on your right foot in a Centering Step.

5. As the hands circle inward and the palms begin to rotate up, the left moves under the right, and then they move together upward in the circling motion so the left hand is underneath the right wrist.

   Both palms face up when they reach chest-height.

   Think opposites. Left leg kicking, right wrist on top. Right leg kicking, left wrist on top.

6. **Your left knee now lifts diagonally to about 4 o'clock without shifting your body weight. As before, your lifted knee locks into the position it reached in the air, before the lower leg extends outward.**

   Think of the knee as a hinge, and flex your foot so you can place a good one on the imaginary opponent to get him (or her) out of your way.

   Avoid locking your knee joint as you lift and extend the leg. This applies to the standing leg, too, because a slightly softened knee gives you more stability.

7. **At the same time as the leg movement, your arms start to lift upward from the shoulders as the wrists rotate, so your palms are facing out. Then your hands separate, palms out, finishing nose-height at about the 5 o'clock and 8 o'clock corners. Eyes follow your left hand.**

Always think about flow. I tell you this over and over. And I won't stop — I'm like a nagging relative. When you practice T'ai Chi, what you are practicing is flow: physical limbs flowing, mental focus flowing, and inner chi flowing.

Now you're a good two-thirds of the way through the Yang-style Short Form. In the next chapter, I finish going over the forms that make up this sequence.

Chapter 11

Closing the Door, Yang-Style

. . . .

. . . .

*W*ith nine forms to go, you can almost see the finish line. But hang on. You've still got a third of the short form to go. And some of the most challenging and varied sequences, too, I might add.

> Right Palm Strike into Snake Creeps Down Left into Rooster Stands on Left Leg
>
> Right Palm Strike into Snake Creeps Down Right into Rooster Stands on Right Leg
>
> Fair Lady Weaves the Shuttle
>
> Pick Up Needle From Sea Bottom
>
> Fan Through the Back
>
> Turn into Backfist down, Parry and Punch
>
> Apparent Close
>
> Crossing Hands
>
> Closing Form

Now, about the favorites in this section:

✔ **Closing:** I like this one. And no, silly, not because getting to this point means that I'm done. I like the feeling of settling down, breathing fully with both feet fully planted, and feeling my hands float back into place. I also like staying in this position and enjoying the feeling of quiet.

✔ **Fair Lady Weaves the Shuttle:** Manny votes for this one — no, not because he just likes the concept of a fair lady, either! This movement gracefully combines lifting the body while also absorbing and redirecting an opponent's punch with the front hand, and then responding with an open Palm Strike with the back hand. Did you catch that challenge to combining yin and yang? Take note: Absorb and redirect. Pull back and strike.

Opening Your Mind to Different Versions

Some T'ai Chi forms differ from the ones you find out about in this book, so this chapter gives you the lowdown on these forms. You see, it's the framework and flow of the following few forms that teachers all over sort of tinker with to create their own variations on a theme.

I say "theme" because the moves aren't so entirely different that they leave you scratching your head and furrowing your brow in confusion. The form may require an extra step here, a repeated move there, a different closing, a lengthened form, or some other vision that suits someone's temperament or movement style. It's like looking at a chicken enchilada plate; you recognize the chicken enchilada even if the recipe is different. If you take a bite, you know that it's a chicken enchilada, even if the spices are varied from what you are accustomed to.

In this chapter, I present a version that Manny learned from his teacher. Manny added an extra transitional Palm Strike to start form Numbers 16 and 17, because he says that he sort of looses his chi there without it. (Here chi . . . here chi . . .) It feels better to him this way. And I must say, something can be said for feeling good.

Making the Final Moves

The final moves present some toughies. For example, as you advance, you squat really low on Snake Creeps Down. But don't be concerned with that at first. For now, just get the positioning while keeping your chi flowing. Squatting down farther — "creeping down" — comes with practice and strength, although how low you may go or how you move in any form always depends on your own body as well as your own abilities and needs. Everyone is built differently, and everyone wants something different from this practice. And that's a good thing.

T'ai Chi is not a competition with anyone except yourself. Still, don't take notes about how low you go on a particular day and don't bemoan your lack of ability to keep well-balanced the last time you practiced. Instead, you should think, "Did I practice as diligently as I could have last time?"

The competition lies within, and if you've practiced today, you've already won.

Completing the Third and Last Part, Yang-Style

This last section of the form holds a selection of techniques, weight shifts, and direction changes representative of the traditional long form. So if you decide to practice the long one, too, knowing these variations can help.

In some versions, you go directly from the Parry and Punch to the Closing. In these cases, you don't do an Apparent Close or a Crossing Hands. You take up the extra steps by doing other repeated forms.

All the basic steps and movements that come up over and over — such as Centering Step, Bow Stance, Empty Step, T'ai Chi Hands, and T'ai Chi Posture — are covered thoroughly with illustrations in Chapter 8. So refer to that chapter when those steps and movements come up.

So now, onward to the Closing of the Door.

Right Palm Strike into Snake Creeps Down Left into Rooster Stands on Left Leg (#16)

Also called Rooster Stands on One Leg or Crooked Whip

What you see with this rather long title in front of it, is one version of many used in this form. As long as you perform this form according to all the principles of proper T'ai Chi practice (see Chapter 7), there is no wrong way to do this sequence. Manny's addition of the Right Hand Palm Strike from Single Whip sets up the Snake Creeps Down (see Figure 11-1). This exercise may help you maintain the flow of chi in your body, as it does for him.

1. **Start in the closing form for Kick with Left Heel (see Chapter 10, Figure 10-6). You face about 6 o'clock with your left heel just having finished the kick to 5 o'clock; your arms are fanned outward to the sides, to 5 and 8 o'clock, respectively.**

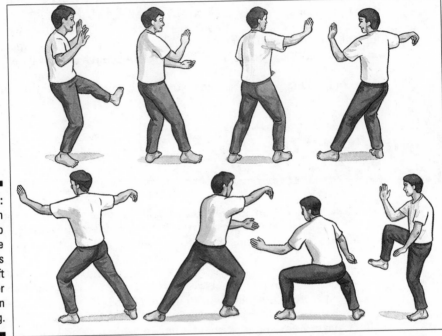

Figure 11-1:
Right Palm
Strike into
Snake
Creeps
Down Left
into Rooster
Stands on
Left Leg.

2. **Here comes the first part, or the Palm Strike: Lower your left foot
   slowly and place it behind your right foot in a stance that isn't as wide
   or as low as a Bow Stance, but is similar. Also rotate your body open
   and turn it slightly toward 7 o'clock.**

3. **Shift your weight back so more of it is over your left foot. At the same
   time, turn your left palm upward and pull the left elbow in to the left
   hip while you press with your right hand over the left palm and push
   away from you, palm out, in the Palm Strike to the front. As you strike,
   shift some of your weight forward again onto a bent right knee.**

   Be sure to keep both elbows soft and not locked. And imagine that you
   are pulling an opponent toward you with the left hand so he is closer to
   strike with the right. Oh, there's that ouch factor again!

4. **Shift your weight again slightly onto your left foot, lift your right toes,
   and rotate the right foot on the heel so the toes face about 8 o'clock.
   Then shift your weight back onto the right foot as you lift your left
   toes and rotate the left foot on its heel so the toes face about 3 o'clock.**

5. **As your feet turn, your body rotates through the waist to face about
   4 o'clock. You again pivot on the right heel to adjust the right toes to
   face 5 o'clock. At the same time, your right arm reaches out toward
   8 o'clock into a Dropped Hand (like in the Single Whip in Chapter 10)
   as the left hand pushes toward 3 o'clock, palm out.**

Avoid locking your knee joint at any time during this maneuvering. And, make sure that when you pivot your feet, you slightly unweight each one so you don't twist your knees.

6. **Snake Creeps Down Left: Rotate the right toes back to 8 o'clock (again, lifting on the heel and pivoting as usual without weight on the foot). At the same time, slowly flip the left palm inward, thumb up, as the forearm hinges from the elbow to sweep the left palm past the face as it turns into a "snake."**

If you are a novice, the wider lunge with right toes to 8 o'clock may feel uncomfortable or awkward. If so, simply rotate the toes inward more (to 5, 6, or 7 o'clock) so the stance is not as wide or turned out. As you become stronger and more experienced, you'll be able to turn the toes out farther.

Keep your right hand in the hooked "dropped" position while the "snake" slithers.

7. **Bend the right knee so you sink toward the ground as far as you can. The left knee extends — but doesn't lock straight — and the toes stay on the ground. Let the left-hand "snake" glide past the body (palm parallel with your body) and down past the front of the right knee to start a circle back up and to the left. As it grazes past the knee, the palm rotates perpendicular to the body, thumb out. The right Dropped Hand follows behind the left arm, down, and then up to the left.**

Make sure that your right knee stays over your right toes (and left knee over left toes) to protect the joint when you bend and sink over each side.

8. **Stay in a crouched position. Begin bending the left knee and extending the right knee as you shift your weight back to the left side.**

9. **Rooster Stands on Left Leg: As you begin to lift out of the crouch to the left, pivot on your heels so your left toes face between about 3 to 4 o'clock and your right toes about 5 o'clock in another Bow Stance facing 3 o'clock. Your right hand has opened out of Dropped Hand and is to your front; your left hand is pushing forward to 3 o'clock.**

10. **Bring your right toes into a Centering Step and straighten the left leg.**

Use this Centering Step, however fleeting, to find your balance in preparation for the next one-legged stance.

11. **Lift your right knee. At the same time, lift your right hand so the elbow is bent and pointing down. The elbow and knee touch briefly at about waist-height. The right hand is perpendicular to your body with fingers facing skyward and thumbs in. Your eyes look through the hand and beyond.**

12. **Lower your left palm so it is now facing down at your left hip.**

What to avoid:

- ✔ Trying to crouch lower than you are able as the "snake creeps down"
- ✔ Turning your feet without shifting your weight to release your toes (so you can pivot easily and not add extra torque on your knee joint)

Right Palm Strike into Snake Creeps Down Right into Rooster Stands on Right Leg (#17)

Also called Crooked Whip, or Rooster Stands on One Leg

This form is a repeat of the previous form on the opposite side. I flip the steps so you get the hang of the form, but you may want to refer to the previous steps for full details. Starting again with the Right Palm Strike on the opposite side may seem odd, but Manny leaves in this movement because the flow seems to work better for him. Give it a whirl and see what suits your fancy. Refer to Figure 11-2 for a visual.

1. **Palm Strike: From the one-legged Rooster position where you end in the previous form, lower your right foot forward into a Bow Stance still facing 3 o'clock. At the same time, allow your left hand to rotate palm up at your hip as if it simply hangs on to that mean ol' opponent so you can whack him with your right hand, which pushes (strikes) forward.**

2. **To continue on the opposite side, refer to Steps 4 through 12 in the previous form. However, this time you pivot your weight, so you now continue to turn yourself around on the clock face in the same direction, opening yourself toward your front at 12 o'clock.**

   Don't forget to pivot on your heels to protect your knees.

3. **Rotate your left toes to 1 o'clock by pivoting on your heel. Your right toes still face about 3 o'clock.**

4. **Shift your weight onto the right foot and bend the right knee. At the same time, push your right hand out to 3 o'clock and lift your left hand down and up to 10 o'clock in the Dropped Hand position (see Single Whip, in Chapter 10).**

   There are a few extra shifts and rocks of your weight here and there, especially in these Snake forms. These were added in this variation to help you gather and build your chi and add power to the coming move, Manny says. Once again, this harks back to the defensive foundation of T'ai Chi — if you're going to do more than just look pretty, you need to find your power and chi.

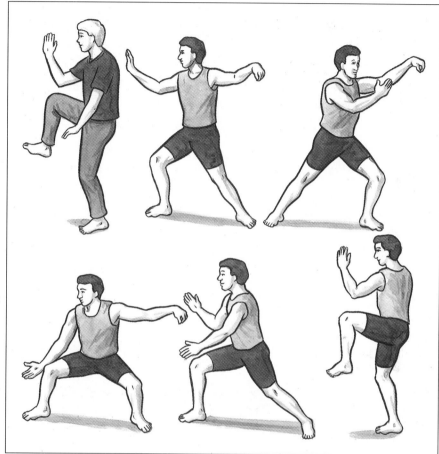

Figure 11-2:
Right Palm
Strike into
Snake
Creeps
Down Right
into Rooster
Stands on
Right Leg.

5. **Snake Creeps Down Right:** The body rotation and arm circling, as
   described in Steps 6 through 8 in Snake Creeps Down Left, are identical, except the left foot now rotates to 10 o'clock to open the hips and
   the right palm becomes the creeping snake that circles past your face.
   It glides down toward your left knee and past your body as you bend
   your left knee, followed by the left Dropped Hand. Then it completes
   the circle back up to the right as you move your body weight over the
   right knee, to the center, and then to the left.

6. You end the right-snake-creeping by rotating your body with your
   arms to 3 o'clock in a continuous sweep. Your right toes pivot on the
   heel to face about 4 o'clock so you are in another Bow Stance with
   your left hand opened out of Dropped Hand and to your front; your
   right hand pushes forward to 3 o'clock.

7. **Rooster Stands on Right Leg: This time, the sweep finishes with the left toes lifting to graze past your right ankle in a Centering Step for balance. Then the left knee lifts up to also point toward 3 o'clock.**

You may need a nanosecond in this Centering Step to reset your alignment and catch your balance. It helps to exhale on the push forward in Step 6, inhale on the Centering Step, and then exhale fully in your one-legged Rooster stance.

8. **Lift your left knee. At the same time, lift your left hand so that your elbow is bent and pointing down. The elbow and knee touch briefly at about waist-height. The left hand is perpendicular to your body with fingers facing skyward and thumbs in. Your eyes look through the hand and beyond.**

9. **Lower your right palm so it is now facing down at your right hip.**

What to avoid:

✔ Having your legs and feet end their part of the movements before the arms do

✔ Locking your knee or elbow joints

Fair Lady Weaves the Shuttle (#18)

Also called Fair Lady Works the Shuttles, Throwing the Loom, or Fair Lady Slides the Shuttle

In the Yang long form, the Fair Lady does her weaving four times; basically, she does one weave to each corner with a 90-degree turn between each corner. In this shorter version, you do one toward the right corner and then one toward the left corner, so you still have one 90-degree turn between them. Figure 11-3 helps you with the zigzagging.

Your power comes from sinking the body weight as you shift your weight forward into the strike.

1. **Start from the concluding stance of the preceding form where the left knee is lifted in the one-legged Rooster facing 3 o'clock.**

2. **Place the left foot down at about 2 o'clock, drawing the right toes beside the left ankle in a Centering Step. At the same time, the arms fold into a Hold Balloon position, left arm on top slightly turned to your right.**

The Centering Steps in this form as well as in both sides of the Snake-Rooster form can be left out after you are better at balance and flow. Then you can flow directly into each position of each form.

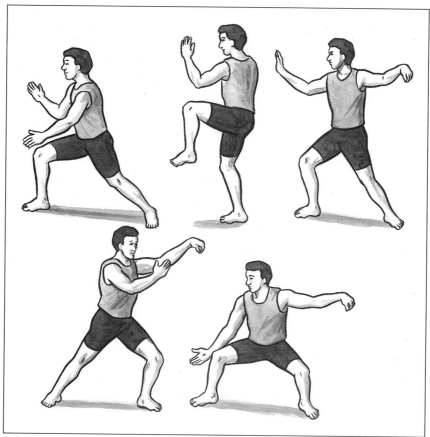

Figure 11-3:
Mirror,
mirror on
the wall,
who's the
Fair Lady
Weaving the
Shuttle?

3. **Inhale and lift the right knee and toe to step into a Bow Stance to 4 o'clock. During this step, lift the right arm, being sure to keep the shoulder relaxed and down. While raising your arm, let the palm turn so the palm ends facing outward and slightly upward at about your forehead; the left hand drops beneath the lifting right arm, pushing out to 4 o'clock with the palm at nose-height, as you exhale.**

This step is where the weaving happens. Just look at your arms.

The lift of the right arm — just as the left arm lift a couple steps from now — should make you feel as if you are blocking someone's approach.

Transition to do the same thing on the other side.

4. **Pull your arms and elbows back and down as you bring your left toes forward next to the right ankle to create a Centering Step on the opposite side, arms in Hold Balloon, right arm on top.**

You still face 4 o'clock. Now, get ready to "weave" again.

5. **Exhale as you step out into a Bow Stance to 2 o'clock, sinking into the left knee, as the arms mirror the arm pattern in Step 3 on the inhale. Lift your left arm, making sure to keep the shoulder down and relaxed and letting the palm turn with the lift so that the palm ends facing outward and slightly upward at about your forehead; the right hand drops beneath the lifting left arm, pushing out to 2 o'clock with the palm at nose-height, again with an exhalation.**

What to avoid:

- ✔ Straightening your knees so you lack power
- ✔ Wandering eyes: Your eyes should follow the pushing and hand weaving under the top arm

Pick Up Needle from Sea Bottom (#19)

Also called Needle at the Bottom of the Ocean, or Needle at the Sea Bottom

You may find that Pick Up Needle is like Strum the Lute (see Chapter 8). That's because you basically shift into an Empty Step using the Bow-to-Empty Step transition that I present in Chapter 8, while your hands move into place. This move is pretty simple, as shown in Figure 11-4.

The main thing to remember on this form is to keep your back straight. Sure, it protects your back, and I'm all about safe movement. But a straight back also helps keep your energy channels open so your chi can easily flow.

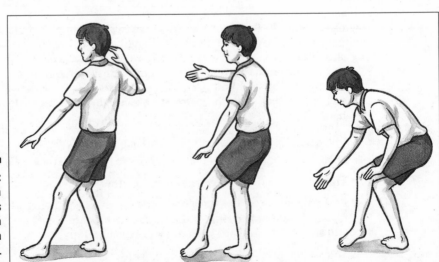

Figure 11-4:
At the Sea Bottom, it's like finding a needle in a haystack.

1. **Start in the last position of Fair Lady, in which you face 2 o'clock in a Bow Stance with the left arm up, palm out, and the right palm pushing out. See Figure 11-3 for details.**

2. **Do another Bow-to-Empty Step transition so you move yourself in one flowing move from one to the other. (See Chapter 8.) As you sit back and sink on the right foot, let your upper body turn from the waist slightly to the right to about 4 o'clock.**

   The next arm movements may remind you of the arms looping around each other and your body in Brush Knee (see Chapter 9).

3. **At the same time that the feet are moving and the body is turning, the arms are also moving. First, the right: The right palm turns to face up and the elbow pulls back behind you, opening your body to almost 6 o'clock as it pulls back. When the elbow is as far back as it can go, continue to hinge open with the forearm, palm up. Then, leaving the elbow high, press forward past your cheek with the right hand. Your body starts to rotate back to 3 o'clock as the right hand brushes past.**

4. **Now add the left arm up to this point: The left palm and elbow turn in and pull across the face and body, reaching to about the right shoulder. Then the left hand circles downward across the front of your torso.**

5. **Here comes the needle part: The right hand, already brushed past your face, now becomes the "needle" as it slices downward to about knee-height, perpendicular to your body and to the inside of your left knee, fingers down. The left hand finishes its circle at your left hip, palm down. You are facing 3 o'clock, and you have exhaled on the last needle-like movement.**

Only go as low as you can with the needle hand (and your back) without pain or discomfort, and be sure to tighten your abdominals to support the back as you lean forward. Consult with your physician about this kind of movement if you have experienced back problems.

What to avoid:

- ✔ Falling forward or putting weight on your left toe when the right needle hand slices downward. (The toe is used only for a touch of balance.)
- ✔ Pulling in your chin to your chest.
- ✔ Straightening either knee.
- ✔ Imagining that the movement ends when you are leaning forward over your knee. (Keep your energy moving and allow it to keep rising to bring you back up.)

Fan through the Back (#20)

Also called Open Arms Like a Fan, or Unfolding Your Arms Like a Fan

Think of making a large fanning motion as you complete this step, shown in Figure 11-5. Also try to engage your back muscles to move your arms through the circling pattern (note the name, "through the back"). Using your back muscles connects the arm movement to your body and better grounds you.

One more thing to imagine about the form in Figure 11-5: An opponent in front of you and one to your left. As you open your arms outward, you deflect each one with a different arm. That's good enough for Hollywood!

1. **Start in the final position of Pick Up Needle (see the previous form) in which you are in an Empty Step with the left foot forward and right hand sliced down to about your knee.**

2. **Lift your upper body and step forward into a Bow Stance to 3 o'clock.**

3. **At the same time, bring up your right arm by bending the elbow and sweeping the hand outward, palm out, in a circular motion in front of your head, ending with it near your right temple as if protecting your head. Your body rotates slightly to 4 o'clock with the movement.**

4. **While your right arm fans up and around protecting your head from an imaginary opponent, your left arm also lifts upward and outward, palm out. It finishes at about nose-height, toward 3 o'clock.**

Let your gaze follow your left, forward-fanning hand.

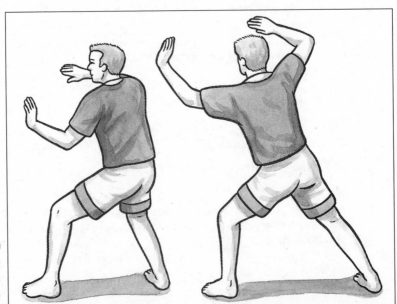

Figure 11-5:
Fan, fan, fan
we go.

What to avoid:

- Placing your left arm and left leg on different planes
- Making the Bow Stance too wide for a powerful block
- Bending your knee so deeply that it pokes beyond your foot and the joint doesn't get proper support

Turn into Backfist Down, Parry and Punch (#21)

Also called Turning Around, Warding Off, Punching; or Deflect Downward, Parry and Punch; or Strike Parry and Punch

You want a strong punch? Do it with a fist held in T'ai Chi style, although in T'ai Chi, you are primarily working on your mindful energy flow, not your immediate ability to punch and sock. With a T'ai Chi Fist, the curled fingers face in, so if you open the fist, you look like you are ready to karate chop a stack of phone books (or, for a friendlier analogy, like you're ready to shake somebody's hand). The wrist aligns with the forearm (not cocked to the right or left) so the bones in the lower arm are placed in their strongest position. Less chance of wrist buckling, too. Oh, and this fist is called a "vertical fist" because the palm is in a vertical position. You can see it in Figure 11-6.

The name of the move includes the word "backfist" because you hold your right fist to block downward against the opponent. But you can also try this with a "hammer fist" by holding the butt of your palm — that's the fleshy part where it meets the wrist — downward, which is something that Manny sometimes likes to do. You may see different looks of this move too, depending on teachers, style, and taste.

Variety is the spice of life, right? That and having an open enough mind to try something different, maybe just to see how it feels.

1. **Start in the concluding position of the Fan. That means in a Bow Stance facing 3 o'clock with arms spread up and out. Refer to Figure 11-5 for positioning.**

   Now you get to do nearly a full pivot to your right from 3 o'clock

2. **Shift your weight back onto your right foot so you can pivot your left toes to face about 7 o'clock. Then place your weight back on your left foot — bending your knee of course — so you can draw your right toes in to graze your left ankle in a Centering Step facing 8 o'clock but with your body turned through the waist to 9 o'clock.**

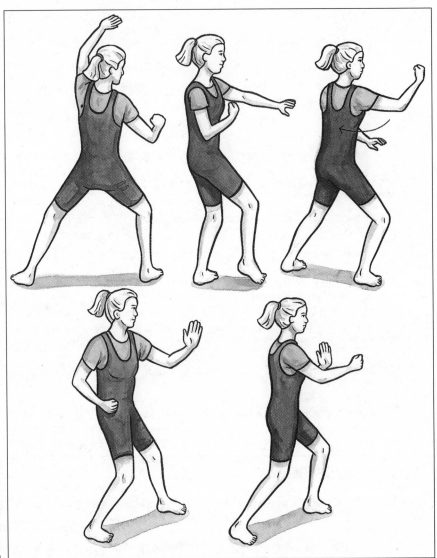

Figure 11-6:
Turn into
Backfist
Down, Parry
and Punch.

3. **Your arms also need to gather in toward you as you pivot:** Your right
   arm pulls down to your right side, palm in, as your left arm rolls up
   and over, palm out. The left arm ends up swinging somewhat over
   your head as you pivot so it ends palm out, in front of you, also to
   8 o'clock. The right arm at your side bends at the elbow, lifting up to
   the front of your abdomen as the hand turns into a T'ai Chi Fist, fingers to body.

Refer to Chapter 8 for some hints on making a T'ai Chi Fist. For now, try this one fingers in and palm up.

4. **Backfist Down: Continue to move your backfist up along your chest (in kind of a windup for a good whack on the opponent with the back of your fist) as your left arm moves down to your side.**

   The right fist now lifts up to about nose-height and pulls straight down to 9 o'clock on its way to being pulled into your right hip, fingers up but still in a fist. Exhale on the backfist-down move.

5. **Parry: At the same time, step out a little with your right foot, placing your weight on the heel and, as you roll onto the foot, allow the toes to pivot to face about 11 o'clock. Your left hand has floated back up your left side and the palm pushes out to about 10 o'clock at the same time the backfist pulls in to the right hip, fingers up.**

   You inhale on this move.

   Don't forget to bend your right knee as you roll your weight onto it.

6. **Your left foot, now unweighted, draws into a brief Centering Step for balance (if needed) and then is placed out into a Bow Stance to 8 o'clock with toes facing 9 o'clock.**

7. **Punch: Roll your weight back onto the left leg, bending the knee in a Bow Stance, allowing yourself to fully sink into the knee. At the same time, the left arm pushes out to about 10 o'clock at chest-height, and the right arm punches out in a "vertical fist" to 9 o'clock just to the right of the left hand.**

   Here, you exhale again for additional power.

Let the punch come not only from your arm, but also from the connection all the way up from your right heel. ***Remember:*** "United we stand" — unite your entire body to let that imaginary opponent fall and your energy flow.

What to avoid:

- Rotating without lifting your toes or without unweighting the foot, which puts undue strain on the knee joint
- Holding your breath

Apparent Close (#22)

Also called Closure

Here I am, all the way at the end, and you get to see a true T'ai Chi defensive principle in practice: If you want to push away your opponent, first pull the ol' meanie toward you. That's what you do when you "apparently" close (see Figure 11-7). Then, when he starts to pull back, you just help him out a little. Tricky, tricky.

1. **From the closing position of Backfist Down, you are in a Bow Stance with the right fist punched forward and the left hand pushed out over it with the palm.**

2. **Let the left hand "sneak" under the right forearm by tipping the fingertips down and snaking the top of the fingers and the back of the hand under the forearm. Open the fist of the right hand.**

3. **At the same time, start to sit back on the right leg. Turn both palms up and separate the hands at chest-height; then pull the elbows toward your waist. Turn both palms down when they reach your body.**

   When you sit back, let the left knee bend and extend the left leg, also lifting the left toes a little off the ground.

4. **Without interrupting the flow, let your weight return to your left leg and push forward with your palms, all toward 9 o'clock.**

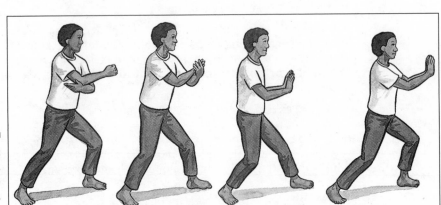

Figure 11-7:
Apparently,
we're
closing now.

Crossing Hands (#23)

Start the close with this simple hand-crossing form, shown in Figure 11-8. Aim for slow and smooth, so you don't lurch, grind, and stutter to a stop. This is another part of the closing forms that differs among schools and styles.

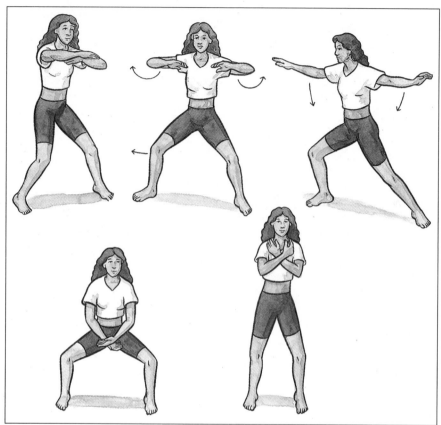

Figure 11-8:
Cross your
hands and
hope to . . .

1. From the final push position of the Apparent Close, begin again to rock your weight back onto your right leg.

2. At the same time, bring your hands in and cross them in front of your body at about the wrist with the right arm closest to your body. The hands are placed at about chest-height.

3. Next is a Sweep Open transition, as I describe in Chapter 8. Pivot to return to the front to face 12 o'clock by lifting your left toes and turning on the heel and then replacing the toes to the ground to face 12 o'clock. Shift your weight back to the left leg so you can then pivot your right foot and toes to also face 12 o'clock.

4. At the same time, slide your hands over the forearms and apart, reaching out to each side, palms down.

Your eyes should follow your right hand, as if you think some opponent is hiding on the right side ready to pounce.

5. **During this movement, step out wide to the right with your right foot, toes turned out to 2 o'clock. Arms drop down as you bring your weight back to the center, and then do a little squat by bending both knees a little.**

6. **During the squat, your hands scoop down in front of your body from their wide position and then pull inward in front of your torso to cross again at the wrists, palms in, right arm on top before it again pulls in closest to your body.**

Be sure to keep your chest lifted and back straight when you scoop to the front. Tight abdominals also protects your back. Modify this move if you have back problems and be sure to consult a physician.

7. **At the same time that you pull the arms in, shift your weight to your left leg and pull your right leg underneath you, toes pointed forward and feet about hip-width apart.**

What to avoid:

- ✔ Locking your knees when you return to face forward with feet hip-width apart
- ✔ Rounding your back forward on the squat and the arm-circling movement

Closing Form (#24)

Also called Closing the Door or Conclusion

Don't just do the form and then run off to make dinner or answer the telephone! Enjoy this closing form as a satisfying way to finish your practice. Stay still in this final stance for a few moments, take some deep breaths, and let your weight sink into the roots of your feet and into the earth. Figure 11-9 shows you how.

You may find more variations here between teachers in areas such as knee-bends, timing, or stepping. Choose what feels right to you.

1. **Start in the closing position of Crossing Hands with feet centered, toes facing forward and hands crossed in front of your chest, and slowly inhale.**

2. **Exhale, and slowly uncross your wrists by turning palms in and down; then slide the left hand over the top of the right and both hands down.**

3. **Float your hands to your sides. Palms lead downward until the hands and wrists are extended and at your side.**

4. **Using good T'ai Chi Posture (see Chapter 8), palms face in to your thighs. Inhale, sink into your knees and letting them bend, and then exhale and return to a standing position.**

If you want, you can also bring your feet closer together in the final position (Step 4) as your lift upward from a bent-knee position: Just step in. Experiment with both feet to find what's most comfortable to you.

If going through the Yang-style short form only whets your appetite, you may want to take a look at the longer version of this form. Performing the long form can pay you back many more times the amount of time and effort you spend on it. On the other hand, if you are content with the short form that I present as an introduction to T'ai Chi, that's fine too. Continue to work on it, and be aware of all that your body feels as it flows along.

No form initially reveals all of its gifts to your mind and body. Beginning to practice the forms is like reading Shakespeare. As a young person, it was sort of confusing and perhaps a bit odd to boot. But the more you read it, the more you understood some of the subtle meanings and what was going on. This short form, like one of Shakespeare's works, may seem odd at first dabble, but you'll learn to love it as it becomes a mainstay of a lifelong study. Learn it, take it apart a piece at a time, refine it, understand it, and let it lead you to yourself.

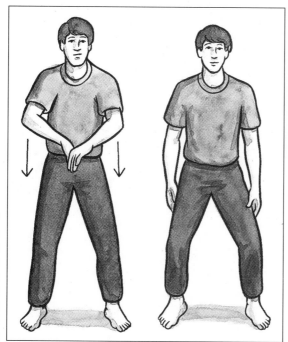

Figure 11-9: Not just apparently closing. It's almost really time to go!

Chapter 12

Trying Out Manny's Short Form

• •

In This Chapter

▶ Using simpler forms

▶ Getting information from Manny

• •

*I*n the world of T'ai Chi, there are a lot of versions of forms, short and long. Even the "short" forms can be pretty long and darn challenging, especially for novices, seniors, and people rehabilitating from any injuries or suffering from any chronic pain disorders, even the likes of low back pain. That's the reason Manny's Short Form was born.

If you want a stepping stone to help you master the whole Yang Short Form (see Chapters 9 through 11 for that step-by-step sequence), read on. Manny's Short Form can be yet another form in your T'ai Chi bag o' tricks to keep you challenged as you mix and match your practice.

Forms you see in this chapter:

> Opening Move
>
> Ward Off — Left
>
> Grasp the Bird's Tail — Right
>
> Sweep the Table — Left
>
> Grasp the Bird's Tail — Left
>
> Sweep the Table — Right
>
> Single Whip
>
> Wave Hands Like Clouds — Right
>
> Listen to Seashell — Left Ear
>
> Repulse the Monkey
>
> Figure Eight, Drop, Gather
>
> Fair Lady Weaves the Shuttles — Left and Right
>
> Single Whip

Wave Hands Like Clouds — Left

Listen to Seashell — Right Ear

Repulse the Monkey

Windmill

Closing

Using another T'ai Chi Short Form

Manny's version isn't just some hybrid form of T'ai Chi that doesn't look or feel like real T'ai Chi, as some contemporary mind-body practices are. This is *real* T'ai Chi, with the same forms used in Yang, but fewer of them, more repetitions, and with some of the harder ones left out.

Manny's creation is a good introduction to T'ai Chi form practice. You have the chance to use all the principles of good T'ai Chi (see Chapter 7 for more on principles), such as moving slowly and breathing fully. You just have less to boggle your brain.

This form should take about 4 to 5 minutes to practice if you learn it. So you may want to do two or three of them in a row after you can make your way through the pieces without having to stop and flip pages every step or two. This gives you about 10 to 15 minutes of good practice.

The origin of Manny's form

As told by Manny himself: This form came into being in 1994. John, a physical therapist at the hospital where I worked, brought me an article from a scientific journal that reported some studies on preventing injuries in seniors. The article was called "Frailty and Injuries: Cooperative Studies of Interventional Techniques," sponsored by the National Institutes of Health. (See the Appendix for a complete reference.)

This large-scale study looked at the effectiveness of eight different ways to prevent falls in seniors. The findings reported that T'ai Chi was the most effective prevention used in the study.

With that kind of solid information about T'ai Chi's benefits, I got permission from my administration

to start a class for the seniors of the community. To prepare for the class, I began to look around to determine which of the many T'ai Chi forms and exercises would be best for the older beginner. Despite all the great forms, I didn't find any forms that had everything I was looking for. So I devised my own! I based it on movements from the Yang Short Form.

For four years, I taught this form successfully to seniors, and my classes grew. I now work at a different hospital, and I use my form to teach T'ai Chi not only to seniors but also to the beginning public and to participants in the Pain Management Clinic at my hospital.

Stepping up to a simpler short form

Like everything in life, you get out of T'ai Chi what you put into it. Longer forms mean longer practice and, therefore, greater benefits. But Manny understands the demands of today's society, so he created this shorter, simpler short form. And you still get a good dose of health benefits (see Chapter 2).

All but 6 of the 18 forms in Manny's Short Form are identical to ones in the Yang 24-Movement Short Form. (I put an asterisk by the ones that are new so you can pick them out.) And of those six, two of them repeat, so you only have four entirely different movements. In the other cases, the forms are pure Yang, but they are positioned differently, used only in part, presented once instead of two times or more, done multiple times instead of once, or transitioned a little differently.

You may note one difference: Some forms are done not only on the same side as in the Yang Short Form, but they're also done on the opposite side! Yikes, mirror-image stuff, which can be difficult for the brain to catch first time out of the gate. Manny created this style because he felt that the students who took his class typically needed to work on both sides equally for better muscle and balance training. In the Yang Long Form, both sides of each form are already included.

Taking On Manny's Short Form

You'll see a lot of forms, but you may already be familiar with the other forms from Chapters 9 through 11. So Manny's form is not really so new.

I provide instructions and figures in Chapters 9 through 11 for the forms that are in the Yang Short Form series. When these forms come up in this chapter, I describe any necessary transitions and then refer you to the appropriate chapter and figure so you can flip back easily. For the new forms, I present all the instruction here. However, if the form is on the opposite side, I provide instruction so you can work through it more easily.

For the how-to on transitions, basic stances, hands, arms, and posture, take a look at Chapter 7.

Opening Move (#1)

Although a seemingly innocuous move, the Opening Move is something you can spend hours on before you even entertain the idea of moving on. In fact, that is often recommended by T'ai Chi masters, partly because in this little two-step, you have to practice so many principles — sinking into your knees, feeling your chi, breathing fully, turning your mindful focus inward, and so on. When you catch this form and get your chi flowing, you know it. So don't ask. Just feel.

This Opening Move is the same as the Yang Short Form Commencement. See Figure 9-1 and the corresponding instructions in Chapter 9.

Ward Off — Left (#2)

This move is a teaser for the next movement. Actually, you do a short version of the first part of Grasp the Bird's Tail, which is called "ward off." This move is very "yang" — not as in Yang, the style, but yang, part of yin-yang (see Chapter 3). Basically, Ward Off is an offensive or threatening move. It sort of says, "You talkin' to me? Don't come near! Get outta here!" Refer to Figure 12-1.

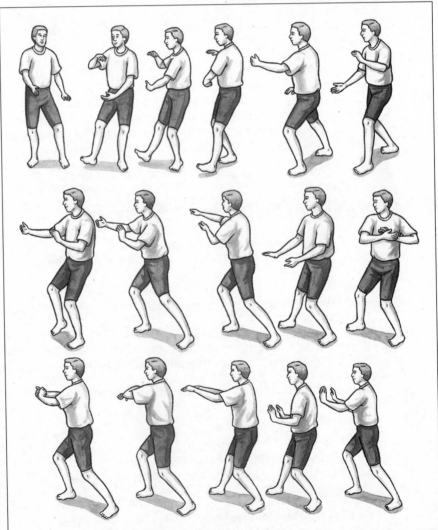

Figure 12-1:
Ward Off —
Left.

1. **Start in the closing position of the Opening Move, still facing 12 o'clock in a stance with feet hip-width apart.**

2. **Begin to lift your right hand forward slightly as if you are getting ready to shake somebody's hand in front of you. Before you get the hand to a hand-shake height, however, rotate the right hip open to 3 o'clock by lifting the right toes and pivoting on the heel so the toes are placed back on the ground facing 3 o'clock.**

3. **As you turn your body, lift the right hand up to chest-height and turn the palm down, and lift the left hand upward so the palm is below the right and facing upward toward it, as if you were holding a ball of energy in front of you.**

4. **Your right knee bends more as you rotate your body fully to 3 o'clock. At the same time, bring your left toe briefly past your right ankle in a Centering Step (see Chapter 8); then continue its movement outward into a Bow Stance (see Chapter 8) with left toes facing about 1 o'clock.**

If you feel well-balanced, you can leave out the Centering Step and bring your left foot directly out into the Bow Stance. If you do use the Centering Step, remember to keep your weight well-balanced and grounded over the right foot. You should be able to do a little heel-toe jig with your left foot and stay rooted on the right foot without shifting your weight.

5. **At the same time that you are moving your weight onto the left foot and bending into the left knee, extend the left hand in front of you with the palm cupped and facing you at chest-height. Point your thumb upward so the elbow is dropped slightly. Your right hand drops palm down at your right hip. You should be facing 3 o'clock.**

What to avoid:

- ✔ Locking your elbows or knees in any part of the move
- ✔ Placing part of your weight on the lifted toe of the Centering Step

Grasp the Bird's Tail — Right (#3)

This form covers the key ingredient to any form — the combination of Ward Off, Roll Back, Press, and Push. The beauty of this four-step form is how the movement flows from *yin* (yielding) to *yang* (aggressive) several times during the sequence. Grasp the Bird's Tail is a great way to get the feel for shifting your weight from one leg to the other.

This form is the same as Grasp the Bird's Tail in the Yang Short Form (see Chapter 9, Figure 9-7).

1. **Start in the final position of Ward Off so your left foot is facing 1 o'clock.**

 2. **Shift your weight completely forward onto your left foot. At the same time, bring your right foot past your ankle in a grounded Centering Step (only if you need to reassure yourself of balance). Then continue the right foot outward to about 4 o'clock in a Bow Stance.**

 3. **Follow Steps 3 through 9 of Grasp the Bird's Tail in Chapter 9, using Figure 9-7 to guide you.**

Sweep the Table — Left (#4)

So this form has a fancy-sounding name. But really, Sweep the Table is just a transitional movement to set up Grasp the Bird's Tail on the left side. (See Figure 12-2.) Still, don't minimize the importance of transitional movements! You should still perform them with the same focus that you perform the other movements. Why is this form called Sweep the Table? Imagine being in a hurry to clear the dining table and brushing everything off in one full sweep. Reminds me of the White Rabbit's tea party in *Alice's Adventures in Wonderland,* only messier.

 1. **Start in the final position of Grasp the Bird's Tail, where you are facing 4 o'clock in a Bow Stance in the Push position.**

 2. **Turn both palms down and "sweep" them together across the front of your body to your right. They are still at chest-height. Move them as far to your right as you can, or to about 10 or 11 o'clock.**

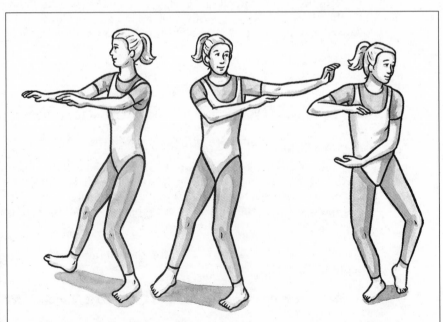

Figure 12-2:
Sweep the
Table —
Left.

3. **At the same time, let your right toes follow your hands; pick up your right toes and pivot the right foot on the heel until the toes can be placed back on the ground facing about 12 o'clock.**

   Be sure to keep the left knee bent and over the toes, instead of wobbling back and forth, which can strain the knee joint.

4. **Shift your weight back onto the right foot, and bring your left toes into a Centering Step grazing your right ankle. Your hands move from the forward sweep to a Hold Balloon position (see Chapter 8) with the right hand on top. You now face 12 o'clock again.**

What to avoid:

✔ Torquing your knees farther than the rotation of your toe placement

✔ Letting your knees wobble or extend past your toes in a straining position

Grasp the Bird's Tail — Left (#5)

This movement is the same as Grasp the Bird's Tail — Right, the third movement in this chapter, but on the opposite side. (See Chapter 9, Figure 9-7 for an illustration of it in the Yang form.)

1. **Start in the final position of Sweep the Table. Adjust your right foot as you move into the first Ward Off position so it points between 10 and 11 o'clock (about 10:30) rather than straight ahead. Do this by pivoting on the heel.**

2. **Follow Steps 2 through 10 of Grasp the Bird's Tail in Chapter 9, using Figure 9-7 to guide you.**

To avoid tightening up your back or twisting your knee, be sure to make the foot adjustment to the right side in the first move.

Sweep the Table — Right (#6)

Another repeat! Isn't this form fun? This is the same as the table-clearing gesture in Figure 12-2, but on the opposite side. You gotta stay balanced, right? Refer to Figure 12-3 for this move.

1. **Start in the final position of Grasp the Bird's Tail, where you are facing 8 o'clock in a Bow Stance in the Push position.**

2. **Turn both palms down and "sweep" them together across the front of your body to your left. They are still at chest-height. Move them as far to your left as you can, or to about 1 or 2 o'clock.**

3. **At the same time, let your left toes follow your hands. Do this by picking up your left toes and pivoting the left foot on the heel until the toes can be placed back on the ground facing about 12 o'clock.**

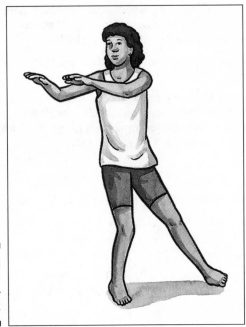

Figure 12-3:
Sweep the
Table —
Right.

4. **Shift your weight back onto the left foot, and bring your right toes into a Centering Step grazing your left ankle. Your hands move from the forward sweep toward your body, palms facing in, about 6 inches apart, in front of your navel as if you are holding a much smaller ball of energy. You now face about 11 o'clock.**

Single Whip (#7)

This movement is the same as the Single Whip in the Yang Short Form, but on the opposite side. Refer to Figure 12-4 for this form.

To set up this move, imagine that you are pulling a ball of energy into your midsection and then letting it flow out into your hands as you settle into the Single Whip form with a Dropped Hand. (For more information on the Dropped Hand, see Figure 8-6 in Chapter 8.)

1. **Start in the final position of Sweep the Table in the preceding form, or in a Centering Step with your weight over your left foot, which points to about 12 o'clock.**

2. **Step outward to about 4 o'clock with the side of your right foot, but the toes face 3 o'clock. Allow your torso to rotate to 12 o'clock as you float the left hand to your side (to about 10 o'clock) into a Dropped Hand. At the same time, your right hand floats upward in front of your chest, finishing palm in. The left elbow is also bent and dropped downward slightly.**

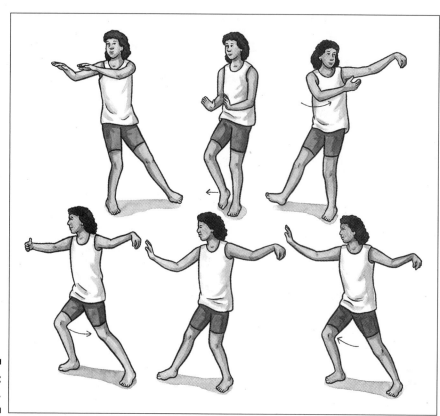

Figure 12-4:
Single Whip.

No move truly "finishes," although I sometimes use that word. I just mean that a position described at that moment is one you see before moving onward to the next transition and the next form.

3. **Shift your weight onto your right foot and let the torso and hands move over the right foot with you. Move as far as you can without forcing yourself. As you shift to the right, let your left foot pivot on the heel so the toes turn inward slightly to point to 1 or 2 o'clock.**

Adjusting the foot helps take any possible pressure off the back or knees. Feel free to make adjustments in other forms, too, if you feel that a particular foot or arm position doesn't feel good to your body. Don't worry, the T'ai Chi gods won't strike you with lightning for it! They want you to feel good, too.

4. **Turn to face 3 o'clock, moving your arms to follow the torso's movement; the left dropped hand now reaches to between 10 and 11 o'clock (10:30 if you're keeping score), and the right curved hand is blocking anyone coming at you from 3 o'clock.**

5. Shift your weight to sit back onto the left leg as you relax the right arm, letting the right elbow drop down and the hand turn palm down as if you are sliding the palm down toward you over the top of a ball. Finally, your hand, palm out, flows back over the top of the imaginary ball as you push your weight and palm back forward to 3 o'clock.

Wave Hands Like Clouds (#8)

Manny really loves to wave his hands around! And you can tell here since this form is not only repeated four times, but is also done later on the opposite side another four times! That means you get to fully practice inhaling when you shift your weight, and exhaling as you close together with your feet.

This form is the same as the Yang Short Form version. (See Figure 10-2 in Chapter 10.)

1. **Start in the final position of Single Whip in the preceding form.**

2. **Your right hand scoops down to about navel-height, and the left palm opens as you shift your torso to face 12 o'clock. At the same time, your left foot pivots on the heel to also face 12 o'clock again.**

   Now you're ready to start the smooth hand-waving and side-stepping of Wave Hands.

3. **Follow the instruction in Chapter 10, Wave Hands Like Clouds, Steps 2 through 7, except move to the right instead of the left: Drop your left hand downward as you shift your weight to your right foot; then bring your left foot to join it. Repeat this side-stepping motion four times by reaching out with your right foot as you drop the left hand and lift the right hand.**

4. **Finish with your feet parallel, left hand lifted, torso turned ever so slightly to the left, and your weight shifted to your left foot. You are facing about 11 o'clock.**

Listen to Seashell — Left Ear (#9)

I'm not sure whether T'ai Chi masters centuries ago listened to seashells. But Westerners get this analogy. You want to feel as if you're holding a really giant — and I do mean *giant* — seashell to your ear to hear the ocean. Refer to Figure 12-5.

1. **Start in final position of Wave Hands Like Clouds in the preceding form, with the left hand lifted to your side, right hand at mid-torso reaching across your body, and your weight shifted onto your left foot.**

2. **Step out with your right foot so your toes face 3 o'clock and shift your weight back to the right foot, letting the knee bend powerfully.**

3. **Sweep your hands across the front of your body, bringing the left arm below the right one and turning the palms so left faces up and right faces down.**

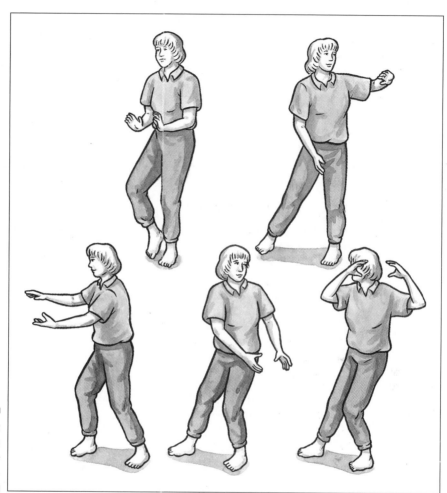

Figure 12-5:
Listen to
Seashell —
Left Ear.

THERESE'S TWO CENTS

You may notice that palms often face each other in sweeping forms like this one. That's because it's a great way to catch your chi.

4. **Finish the weight-shift facing 3 o'clock with your hands capturing the ball of energy in front of your chest.**

5. **Step the left foot toward 12 o'clock and rotate the toes during the step so they face 2 o'clock when the foot lands on the floor again. Your feet are in a smaller Bow Stance.**

6. **Keep holding the ball of energy between your hands and float it downward and then up and out toward 12 o'clock. At the same time, spiral your torso and let your weight shift onto the left foot.**

7. **Continue circling your hands up to the left ear. (Ah-ha! The seashell listening begins!) At the same time, your torso spirals back to face 3 o'clock, and your hands are open to 12 o'clock.**

Repulse the Monkey (#10)

There is no difference between this form and the one you find in the Yang Short Form (see Chapter 9 and Figure 9-6), except that you start facing 180 degrees in the other direction, or toward 3 o'clock rather than 9 o'clock. You step back four times — right, left, right, and then left. Watch this last left step, though. It is slightly different from the Yang model to help you get into the next form.

1. **Start in the final position of Listen to Seashell in the preceding form.**

2. **Let the high right elbow straighten in front of you, keeping the right palm up. At the same time, the right foot steps back behind you, letting the toes touch first and then rolling down through the foot and letting your weight shift onto the right foot.**

3. **As you shift your weight backward, the right elbow pulls in to your waist and then behind it (so your right hand is at the hip, palm up), and the left hand pushes in front of you at chest-height.**

4. **To continue, follow Steps 2 through 6 of Repulse the Monkey in Chapter 9, using Figure 9-6 to guide you. Remember that you are facing the opposite direction, so the first time you open your torso it will be to 6 o'clock with the right hand pulling behind you to 8 o'clock.**

   When you shift your weight backward, the front foot pivots so the toe points straight ahead. But when you lift it up to step back, the foot lands slightly turned out with the knee bending over the toe.

5. **On the fourth and last step backward (with your left foot), step a little farther behind you (see Figure 12-6).**

Figure Eight, Drop, Gather (#11)*

Imagine yourself as a chi fairy who releases the energy from your hands (drops), only to pick up fresh energy with your hands from the earth again (gathers) to pull toward your Dan Tien. (See Chapter 13 for a refresher on that term.) Refer to Figure 12-7 for this form.

1. **Start in the finishing position of Repulse the Monkey in the preceding form, with the left foot stepping back but crossed farther behind you.**

2. **When your foot lands, turn out your toe so it lands facing 12 o'clock. Let the turnout of the toe rotate your torso around to the front. Both toes are now facing front again, and the feet are about hip-width apart.**

3. **At the same time, your torso rotates front, your right hand (which is passing your ear) continues its path forward and ends up, palm in, facing the left hand (also palm in) as if you are holding a mysterious ball of energy.**

   Here comes the Figure Eight.

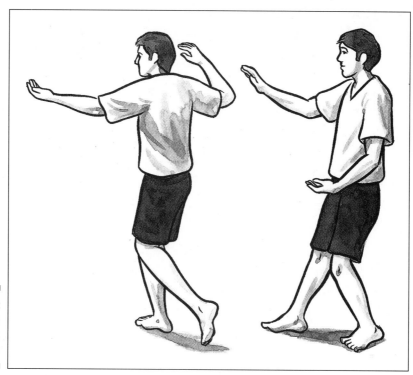

Figure 12-6:
Repulse the
Monkey,
final step.

4. **As your feet turn parallel, drop your hands (but don't drop the ball!) so you are holding the ball in front of your abdomen. Continue the circular pattern, as you swing the ball back up to your left slightly behind your left shoulder as if you want to toss it behind you.**

Let your hips turn slightly with the rotation of your torso and hands so you don't put any pressure on your knees. It should feel natural.

Now you complete the Figure Eight.

5. **Carry your hands (holding the ball) back from behind your left shoulder, drop them toward your middle and down, and then circle them back and over your right shoulder.**

Get ready to Drop.

6. **Let your ball-holding hands drop to the front center. When your torso and hands are at your center, drop your hands and let them separate as they float up to each side (palm down), reaching about waist-height. This move is where you get rid of all the bad chi.**

Now comes the big finale of Gather energy.

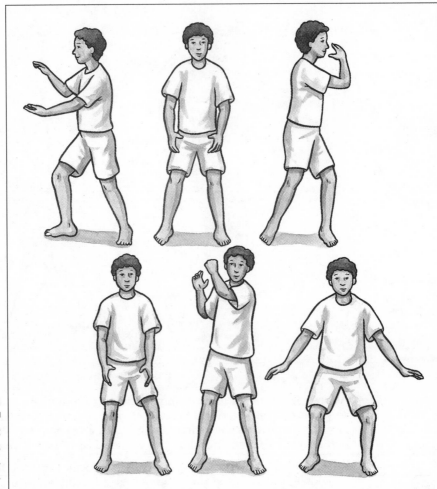

Figure 12-7:
Figure Eight,
Drop,
Gather.

7. **Without truly stopping, the hands go into reverse and float back down again. Here's where you get to scoop up the good chi.**

8. **As you gather up the chi, let your right foot, toes lifted, pivot on the heel so the toes face 2 o'clock. Your left energy-gathering hand turns palm in at chest height, and your right hand is palm up at belly-height as if you are holding a large, tall, very fragile crystal vase next to your torso.**

Keep your right knee bent and your weight sunk into the right leg.

Fair Lady Weaves the Shuttles — Left and Right (#12)

This is the same classic move as in the Yang Short Form (see Figure 11-3 in Chapter 11), except that this move is on the opposite side. I offer some detail here about flip-flopping the steps.

1. **Start in the concluding position of Figure Eight in the preceding form.**

2. **Inhale and step out into a Bow Stance to 11 o'clock with your left foot. During this step, the left arm lifts upward from the shoulder, letting the palm turn with the lift so the palm ends facing outward and slightly upward at about your forehead; the left hand drops beneath the lifting right arm, pushing out to 11 o'clock with the palm at nose-height, as you exhale. (Here's the weaving. See your arms?)**

T'ai Chi's resemblance to a combat martial art shows in the preceding step with the blocking action of the left arm.

Now you just have to transition to do the same thing on the other side.

3. **Pull your arms and elbows back and down as you shift your weight backward onto the right foot, holding your hands as if you are holding a small ball of energy in front of your navel. Lift your left toes when the weight is pulled off; then rock your weight forward onto the left foot. Let the right toes float up next to the left ankle to create a Centering Step on the opposite side, arms in Hold Balloon, left arm on top. You still face 11 o'clock.**

Get ready to weave again.

4. **Exhale as you step out into a Bow Stance to 1 o'clock, sinking into the right knee. The arms mirror the arm pattern in Step 3 on the inhale. The right arm lifts upward from the shoulder, letting the palm turn with the lift so the palm ends facing outward and slightly upward at about your forehead; the left hand drops beneath the lifting right arm, pushing out to 1 o'clock with the palm at nose-height, again with an exhalation.**

Single Whip (#13)

This form is nearly the same move as the Single Whip described earlier in this chapter and the ones in the Yang Short Form. You may note that this one doesn't include all the sweeping of the arms as in the Yang Short Form. So be sure to really use the pushing and retreating of this version. Refer to Figure 12-4, earlier in this chapter.

1. **Start in the concluding position of Fair Lady in the preceding form, facing 11 o'clock.**

2. **Let your weight shift to your left foot while turning your body through the waist to face about 10 o'clock. While the body is turning, lift the right toes and pivot the foot on its heel so the toes turn to face about 10 o'clock, too. At the same time, turn your left palm to face you at about nose-height. Let the right hand relax at the wrist to move into the Dropped Hand position reaching toward 2 o'clock.**

Don't forget to lift the toes for the foot-pivot so you don't twist your knee.

3. **Shift your weight back onto your right foot, sinking into the bent knee. Pull your left hand, palm out, slightly in to your chest in kind of a**

windup (as if you are going to push someone away). **Pull in the left toe to a Centering Step, facing 10 o'clock.**

 4. **Lift your left toe and step outward to about 8 o'clock into a Bow Stance, while your left hand pushes forward, palm out, to about 9 o'clock. (Now you get to push that imaginary person away.)**

Wave Hands Like Clouds (#14)

Here you go, waving your hands again! Enjoy this flowing lateral movement. This one truly repeats the Yang Short version, moving to the left.

 1. **Start in the finish position of Single Whip, in the preceding form.**

 2. **To continue, follow Steps 1 trough 7 of Wave Hands Like Clouds in Chapter 10, using Figure 10-2 to help guide you.**

Listen to Seashell — Right Ear (#15)

This form is a repeat of Listen to Seashell described earlier in this chapter (see Figure 12-5), except on the opposite side. Be sure to give equal attention to both sides.

 1. **Start in the final position of Wave Hands in the preceding form.**

 2. **Step out with your left foot so your toes face 9 o'clock, and shift your weight back to the left foot, sinking into the bent left knee.**

 3. **Sweep your hands across the front of your body to the left, bringing the right arm below the left one and turning the palms so the right faces up and the left faces down.**

 Use the palms facing each other to feel the warmth of your chi as you catch it.

 4. **Finish the weight-shift facing 9 o'clock with your hands capturing the ball of energy in front of your chest.**

 5. **Keep holding the ball of energy between your hands and spiral it downward to the right and then up and out toward 12 o'clock as you rotate your torso with it and let your weight shift onto the right foot.**

 6. **Continue circling your hands up to the right ear. (Time for seashell listening again!) At the same time, your torso spirals back to 9 o'clock so you can be ready to Repulse the Monkey, next.**

Repulse the Monkey (#16)

I think that Manny put this one in again because he likes the name so much. There is something about the thought of repulsing monkeys that makes everyone giggle. Oh, and this one faces and moves the same way as the one you see in the Yang Short Form in Chapter 9.

 1. **Start as you finished in Seashell Listening, in the preceding form.**

2. **To continue, refer to Steps 2 through 6 in Chapter 9. Figure 9-6 can help you. This one starts with a step back with the left foot, however. So the progression here is left, right, left, right.**

Windmill (#17)

This movement may remind you of pieces from two others. The body twists from side to side as in the Figure Eight (see Figure 12-7 in this chapter), while the hands and arms float and sway as in Wave Hands Like Clouds (see Figure 10-2 in Chapter 10). You sway four times, going right, left, right, and then left to finish. Refer to Figure 12-8.

1. **Start in the finishing position of Repulse the Monkey in the preceding form, with the right foot stepping back but crossed farther behind you.**

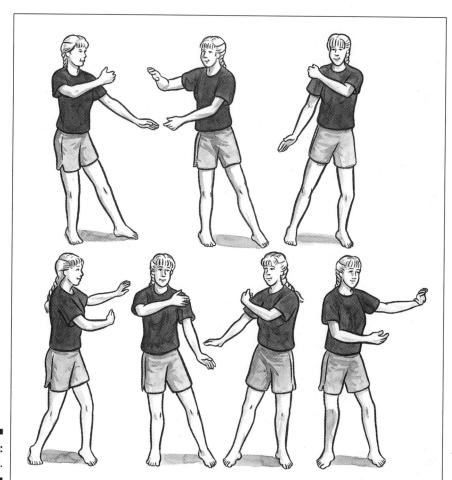

Figure 12-8:
Windmill.

2. **When your foot lands, turn out your toe so it lands facing 12 o'clock. Let the turnout of the toe rotate your torso around to the front. Both toes are facing front again and the feet are about hip-width apart.**

3. **At the same time your torso rotates front, your left hand (which is passing your ear) continues its path forward and around your torso. The right elbow lifts high to carry you to the right.**

This is actually the first "sway" as you start a similar hand-waving pattern as in Wave Hands Like Clouds, Chapter 10, steps 2 through 5. You will do two "sways" with the right arm and hip to the right, alternated with two to the left.

Note two exceptions: First, you stay in one place without the Wave-Hands side-stepping and, second, your arms move to the right first instead of to the left. So, for example, when you sway to the right, the right elbow that is lifted high leads your body in that direction as the hip turns with it and the weight shifts with it. When you rotate back to the left, the left elbow carried high leads with the same hip rotation and weight shift to the left. In both cases, the opposite arms drops downward, just as in Wave Hands Like Clouds, except without the fancy footwork.

Try to feel a bit like a Raggedy Ann doll being tossed around in the wind. Be sure to inhale with one sway and exhale with the next.

4. **On the final sway to the left, sink a little more into your knees and exhale. Move back toward the center as if you were beginning the sway to the right, but instead settle into a center position.**

This is your a transition to Closing, which is the following form.

Closing (#18)

Like Manny's Opening Move, the Closing is also similar to the Yang Short Form closing — the end! Refer to Figure 12-9.

1. **Start in the finishing position of the Windmill in the preceding form. Stop the rotation with your hips facing front. Your right arm lifts slightly to keep the forearm in front of your body. The left arm floats back across your body, coming outside of the right and going into a crossed position at the forearms in front of your chest. Both palms face in. Inhale when you cross the arms.**

2. **Exhale, and slowly lift to a standing position. At the same time, reach to the sky with your hands, uncrossing the arms and letting them circle up, palms up. As they begin to move to your sides, rotate the arms at the shoulders so the palms face down.**

Use the lift to expand your body and inhale fully.

3. **Float your hands back to your sides. Palms lead downward.**

4. **The arms continue their circle to return back to the front of your chest; the right arm is crossed outside the left so you look like an old Egyptian mummy. Your palms face in again.**

5. Slowly uncross your wrists by turning your palms in and down so they sort of twist around each other. Drop both hands to your sides.

6. In the final position, using good T'ai Chi Posture, palms face in to your thighs. Inhale, sink into your knees and letting them bend, and then exhale and return to a standing position.

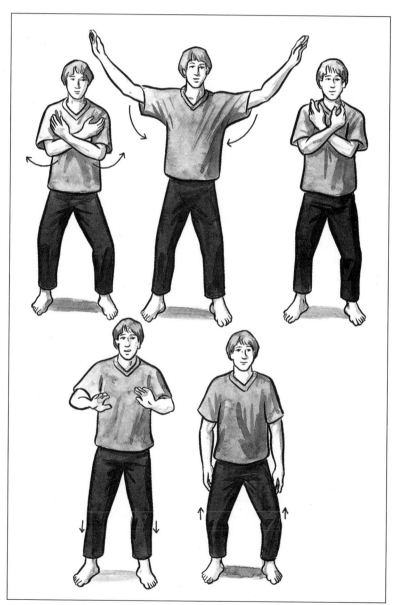

Figure 12-9:
Closing.

Part IV
Energizing Softly with Qigong

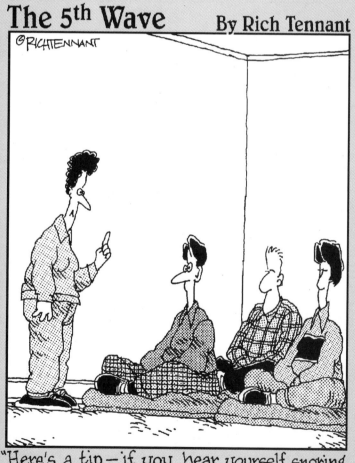

The 5th Wave   By Rich Tennant

©RICHTENNANT

"Here's a tip—if you hear yourself snoring, you're meditating too deeply."

In this part . . .

Qigong is the grandfather of many internal and mindful Asian arts, including T'ai Chi. Its peaceful and chi-stimulating nature makes a wonderful complement to any T'ai Chi practice. In fact, after you read all about the bond between T'ai Chi and Qigong and dive through some of the basic Qigong movements that I present in this part, you may want to find times for doing *just* Qigong. The movements are peaceful and calming, yet energizing and refreshing. These feeling are very different from the ones you get from T'ai Chi, but they're firmly related. So dabble a little and enjoy the differences.

Chapter 13

Recognizing the T'ai Chi–Qigong Bond

- -

In This Chapter

▶ Figuring out what Qigong is

▶ Finding out how to feel the benefits

▶ Meeting your microcosmic orbit

▶ Adding Qigong to your T'ai Chi practice

- -

*H*ey, this book is about T'ai Chi, so why is this Qi stuff suddenly intruding into the T'ai Chi world? Well, my friends, if you believe that T'ai Chi is the ultimate mindful martial art, please sit down. You see, T'ai Chi is actually tightly interwoven with another mindful movement art called Qigong, and it's an important element in a T'ai Chi practice. Qigong is an umbrella term for perhaps hundreds of types of soft methods — both dynamic and still — meant to arouse and free your chi flow. As I explain in Chapter 6, some people go so far as to say that T'ai Chi itself is a complex form of Qigong. Other purists disagree, believing that they are separate and distinct mindful arts. But does that really matter as you try to develop a practice?

Qigong and T'ai Chi are like salt and pepper, bread and butter, Tom and Jerry, or Mutt and Jeff. Wait, I digress. Long story short: They go together like peas in a pod. Some practitioners maintain that you cannot truly and effectively practice T'ai Chi without some infusion of Qigong practice. That's because Qigong works exclusively on developing the internal force and working on your energy flow that is a necessary foundation for an effective T'ai Chi practice.

Deciphering Qigong's Meaning

First things first — you probably want to know what this name means and how the heck you pronounce it. *Qi* (pronounced *chee*) is the more accurate spelling of the Chinese term *chi* or energy (also called "life energy"). Both words are pronounced the same way. *Gong* (pronounced *gung*) means "work" or "a practice," something through which you gain benefits by dedication and practice. Combine the two words and you get "Qigong" *(chee-gung).*

In the Western Hemisphere, the name can also be spelled "chi kung" or even "chi gong," "chi gung," or "chi kung." Some people argue that one or the other is wrong. However, you'll see all of these variations, so recognize that they're all really the same thing. No matter which spelling, the concept of chi is always right up front. For more information on chi, take a look at Chapter 3.

I choose to use "Qigong" compared to the more Westernized "chi kung" (or one of its cousins), because you see that way of spelling it quite frequently. But, seemingly in contradiction I suppose, I choose to use the word "chi" rather than "qi," because when used as a separate word, you tend to see the chi spelling more commonly.

Put it all together, and you see that *Qigong* is a discipline that focuses on working on the flow of your life energy through a dedicated practice. However, in this case, the practice can be moving or still.

Historically historical

Many people have at least heard of T'ai Chi, but most of these people don't realize that Qigong is actually an older form of exercise than T'ai Chi. Traces of Qigong have been found in historical pictograms that date back to hundreds of years B.C. Over the centuries, some Qigong practices were influenced by Taoist masters, and Buddhist monks, who created hundreds and thousands of different styles. Of course, none of these styles are truly wrong, just different, like all the different styles and schools of T'ai Chi.

So, if Qigong is so ancient, why have so few people heard of it, and why are even fewer doing it? For a very long time, Qigong was a very secretive practice, passed down in families (even royal ones) from generation to generation and kept mostly behind closed doors, despite permeating Chinese culture. Although more research and practice was done in the mid-1900s, it wasn't until the 1970s that interest blossomed. The Chinese government watched the growth and finally granted its support and approval in 1985. As a part of the government approval, researchers now present results from hundreds of scientific papers at annual Qigong conferences in China and around the world.

Feeling Qigong's Benefits

Energy is what Qigong is all about. Working with your energy. Feeling it. Gaining it. Moving it (while you move or while you're still). And letting it help you feel healthier and happier.

You may sometimes see T'ai Chi dubbed something like "the slow dance of T'ai Chi" or "the dance of T'ai Chi." That may sound quite lovely but denigrates T'ai Chi to nothing but pretty movement. This is where Qigong steps in. If you want more from your T'ai Chi than a lovely dance, Qigong's ability to develop your internal force and chi is a vital part of your practice. Of course, you don't need to do several hours of Qigong a week while you also do several hours of T'ai Chi. Depending on your interest, you can easily incorporate a few minutes of Qigong into the beginning or end of your T'ai Chi session to reap the benefits that you need. After you learn how to tap into your energy, you may find you need less Qigong practice. Or, you may decide you like it so much that you want even more.

Interestingly, Qigong is backed by some of the most scientific research. Although many of the studies lack some of the strict standards enforced in the West, they are credible and worthy of an eye. In fact, as I point out in Chapter 2, results may speak louder than any scientific proof. Nevertheless, if you want to read more about the science behind the health claims, take a look at Chapter 2, where I also explain the Western idea of health and fitness. Other sources in the Appendix can lead you on your own journey into scientific literature if you are technical minded.

The following sections outline several basic benefits you can gain from a regular Qigong practice.

Finding awareness

Your mind discovers how to open up and become more finely attuned to what is happening within you and outside of you, as well as to how these things are connected. You can gain awareness of your health, your body's movement, any tension or stress, particular feelings, or your relationship to the world that you move through. This awareness is the first step in allowing you to take control of anything that may need action, such as releasing stress or healing a disease, and can be key to healthy longevity

Feeling the focus and calm

The meditative, repetitive, and awareness movements, as well as the flowing routines, bring on a sense of calm, peace, and mental clarity that can permeate everything you do in life. Of course, this benefit isn't scientifically proven, but you try it and see. You may become more focused in work, in relationships, in school, and in all interactions. You may become more relaxed (not a space cadet, just calm and clear), and you may be able to deal better with what comes at you day-to-day.

Even the movements that don't move (or hardly move) create calm and focus because of their concentration on developing a healthy flow of chi.

Gaining higher energy

With more awareness of body and mind, and a more focused calm, comes also a higher energy level. And the energy you gain is vibrant and alive, not like the burst you may get from the likes of caffeine or sugar. You carry this energy throughout all you do, long after your Qigong session is over.

Bettering your breathing

Some of this energy development — as well as the awareness and focus — comes from distinct breathing patterns developed and practiced in Qigong. In fact, if you explore further, you may stumble across classes in which you spend a day or more (possibly years) breathing. You may even read stories of Qigong practitioners who began practicing because they had asthma or other breathing problems.

Qigong masters consider regulated and healthy breathing to be the following:

- ✔ **Slender:** Think narrow streams moving in and out of your nose.

- ✔ **Silent:** Concentrate on quiet and easy inhalations and exhalations.

- ✔ **Deep:** Allow your breaths to be full and move deep into your abdomen instead of shallowly moving in and out of your upper chest area.

Attaining the spiritual summit

If you take the awareness, focus, calm, energy, and breathing a step further, you move into the Three Treasures of Life — something that is beyond the scope of this book. This is not a particular religion, so rest easy. It is related to cultivating Taoist principles and does not rely on any worship.

In short, the three treasures are *jing* (essence), *chi* (energy), and *shen* (spirit).

You cultivate jing to develop chi to become shen. Another way to put it? Chi (through Qigong practice) is the bridge that can carry you from the physical (jing) to the spiritual (shen).

Sorting Out Qigong Goals

Qigong is difficult to pin down with one title or goal. You can practice for a long time and always discover something new. Nevertheless, Qigong works to develop three basic areas:

- **Good health:** Also called "medical" Qigong, this practice is a mix of self-healing techniques and meditation. Qigong is a given in the Chinese medical arena, where it is prescribed for ailments as freely as physical therapy is prescribed in the West.

- **Combat effectiveness:** Developing the inner powers cultivated through Qigong leads to more inner and, therefore, external power in combat or martial applications, which can provide an edge over an opponent. (Not as if you'll be fighting anytime soon, but just finding the inner power can help a daily practice.)

- **Higher spirituality:** Perhaps a step beyond most of your goals, Qigong practices can lead you to higher spiritual development and the expansion of the powers of your mind.

Qigong is a bit like developing your inner power of intuition. You have to train yourself to listen and to trust.

Reviewing Practice Principles

Qigong exercise (see Chapter 14) is a series of dynamic postures or forms that flow from one into the other. The practice also includes simple, stand-alone stances where your mind does much of the work to help release your energy, such as standing meditations, self-massage from standing or seated positions, and breathing practices. You can find a smattering introduction to these stances in Chapter 14. Qigong, in this case, can hardly be called exercise in the traditional Western sense, so don't look for that type of movement.

But no matter which type of Qigong or its goal, you most often find an emphasis on breath work, torso and core stabilization, and visualization.

For an introduction to your chi journey, I look at three regulating principles. If you look closely, you find that these three principles — righting, relaxing, and rooting — are not isolated to Qigong, but appear as principles and foundations to a solid T'ai Chi practice, too.

Righting your posture

You can take a look at Chapter 8 for the description of T'ai Chi Posture. The same tenets apply here. The bottom line is, whether you are practicing Qigong sitting, standing, lying down, or moving, getting your posture right helps you get in touch more quickly with the benefits, including better chi flow.

Minding the medical marvels

The Chinese consider ongoing Qigong practice to be one way of keeping disease at bay. The Chinese philosophy is to prevent disease instead of trying to cure it when it occurs. Slowly, ever so slowly, Western healthcare is beginning to accept this concept. The National Institutes of Health, the medical research center funded by the United States government, has a branch devoted to alternative medicine that has begun to fund research into areas like Qigong and meditation. Some health insurance policies now cover such things as acupuncture and massage as well. (See the Appendix for Web sites and other information.)

You may find Qigong practitioners in the East, and some in the West, too, who use transference of their own well-developed Qi to heal disease or injuries in others, or to keep a person healthy. This method is usually part of a treatment program that includes herbal treatments or other medical care, such as acupuncture.

Qigong's application as a form of medical healing does not fall within the scope of this book. If this treatment is something that interests you, consult your physician.

If you don't stand, lie, move or sit correctly, you can create muscle tension or strain, which can kink your energy hose. (See Chapter 3 for information about chi's flow through energy channels; I go over *meridians,* the energy channels, in the section "Meeting Your Microcosmic Orbit," later in this chapter.)

Maintaining a good posture is also key to tapping into your microcosmic orbit, which I also explain more thoroughly in the next section. (In Chapter 14, you can also find an exercise to help clue into your microcosmic orbit.)

Relaxing your muscles

I don't think that I can adequately emphasize the importance of relaxation. It's key to reaping the basic benefits in Chapter 3. But I'm pointing it out again because it pertains specifically to Qigong.

If you aren't relaxed, you again throw a nasty kink into some part of your energy channels, just as if you don't get the posture right. Relaxation isn't just about making your muscles limp water balloons. It's also about relaxing your joints so they can move better. You also need to relax your face, including your jaw. It means letting go to get hold of your chi.

Letting go is difficult for Westerners. I think that not being busy or tense seems to be perceived as a sign of weakness. In the world of fitness, letting your abdomen relax — that is, letting your belly kind of hang out — is considered a sign of being out of shape rather than being perhaps more in control of *when* you can tighten and relax the muscles.

Good and bad stress, which causes tension in the muscles and other tissues, isn't something that you can truly avoid. So the trick is how you deal with it. And dealing with it to achieve soft and relaxed muscles means the development of better Qigong, which in turn means a better T'ai Chi practice. (Take a look at Chapter 16 for more details on incorporating principles like relaxation into your daily life.)

Don't work too hard, contort yourself, or do anything that doesn't feel good or right to your body and mind. Qigong should feel second nature to you. And if a movement doesn't feel second nature the first time, it may feel natural the third or fourth time. If it doesn't feel natural after a few times, consider two things: seeking out some insights from a master on what you can do better (that's the best choice), or eliminating or modifying the posture.

Rooting your body

A key principle of T'ai Chi (see Chapter 7) that also applies to Qigong, *rooted* means feeling strongly in touch with the ground with your entire foot. Why is this concept so important, particularly to Qigong? Unless you're well-rooted, your chi can't flow freely in your body.

Not rooting yourself well gives you a weak base of support, because you can't stand strongly. It doesn't matter how strong the rest of your body is or how well you think the energy churns around your microcosmic orbit (see the following section). If you aren't rooted well, you can topple with the lightest breeze. Think of a grandiose redwood tree. They appear so tall and strong, but they have roots that are quite shallow, which endangers their longevity. Sometimes, a moderate storm can topple them. Imagine yourself as an oak tree with deep and strong roots, rather than a redwood tree with shallow roots.

Meeting Your Microcosmic Orbit

Microcosmic orbit certainly sounds like a term out of the 1960s cartoon, The Jetsons, but please take it more seriously than a cartoon. A *microcosmic orbit* is a path used to create a rushing flow of chi through two of the largest of your energy channels — the one up the front and the one down the back of you. If you look at yourself from the side (refer to Figure 13-1), imagine an oval starting below your pelvic area (called the *Dan Tien,* which you find out about later in this section) and running up the front to the crown of your head (called the *Bai Hui*). The oval continues from the crown of your head down your back and connects below the Dan Tien. When you do microcosmic orbit meditations (see Chapter 14), you're working to free the flow along these super highways, working the energy up the back, and then back down the front. Some practitioners for different purposes may work to free the flow in the opposite direction. Be sure to keep breathing during all the exercises in Chapter 14 to help your energy move.

Your energy isn't just sloshing around under your skin. Qigong practitioners see it moving through different *meridians,* energy channels, which make up a little network of energy superhighways that run throughout your whole body, with certain gathering centers (highway interchanges) and points of access (on- and off-ramps) where energy more readily flows in, out, and around. Figure 13-1 shows these energy channels and their names.

Despite showing you these energy channels, note that some people — ah, another difference in beliefs! — believe that the energy is a more generalized field of vibrations throughout your body, and not just channeled into certain paths.

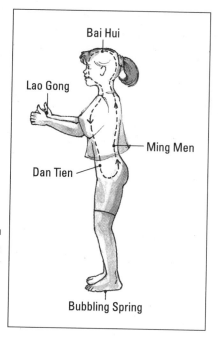

Bai Hui

Lao Gong

Ming Men

Dan Tien

Bubbling Spring

Figure 13-1:
Meet your micro-cosmic orbit.

Circling in on the acupoints

The points of access (the energy superhighway interchanges and on- and off-ramps) are sometimes called *acupoints* because they are also used as gateways in acupuncture. Every spiritual school has different numbers and locations of acupoints, but they all serve the same purpose because they are considered strong and potent areas of the body. Depending on your teacher, he or she may use different names or vary the location slightly.

Dan Tien

The *Dan Tien* (pronounced *don tyen* and literally means elixir field) is akin to NASA's Mission Control for your body's energy, according to Qigong theory. Located between your navel and your pubic bone in the center of your abdomen, the Dan Tien (practice saying this word because you hear it often if you read about or do any Qigong) acts as a storehouse for your body's energy, as well as a pump to get your energy gushing to all the right places when you need it. Doing the right practices and the right movements ensures that you don't lose or gain too much from this center. But this pump needs priming. If you let it sit unused, it dries up. Such practices as Qigong movement, other mind-body methods, and meditation can help prime your pump and keep the chi flowing smoothly.

Late sunrise?

Before I knew a Qigong teacher who was able to answer my questions, I took some classes from an Asian man who spoke little English. He'd say something about a "dawn ten" and sort of point to his belly. I just figured that I couldn't understand what he was saying, shut my mouth, and kept moving. The funny thing was that I actually understood.

As a Qigong student, you may find that nurturing what is underneath an innocent-looking belly becomes a way of life because the elixir field holds long life, health, and wisdom.

See how I spell it Dan Tien? Also look for dantien, dantian, dan-tien, and even tan t'ien in your travels. Don't be alarmed. It's all the same thing. Nevertheless, some purists are promoting standardizing the use of the word to Dantian.

Your Dan Tien has three parts to the command central:

- **Lower Dan Tien:** Located in your lower abdomen and stores sexual energy.

- **Middle Dan Tien:** Located in your center at about your heart and relates to the health of your internal organs.

- **Upper Dan Tien:** What some Eastern practices call the *Third Eye Chakra*. This is the spot on your forehead between your eyebrows and is logically associated with the brain.

If someone says Dan Tien without qualifying the location, they mean the belly area, or the lower Dan Tien.

Ming Men

The term Ming Men was also used by my barely English-speaking instructor. I strained to hear it each time, rolling it around in my brain, trying to figure out what he meant. Turns out, I heard this one right, too. I didn't know what he meant when he said "ming men" and rubbed his lower back.

Literally meaning "gate of life," the Ming Men (pronounced *ming mun*) acupoint controls your kidneys and is located in your lower back. If stimulated properly, Ming Men keeps the kidneys functioning well and can increase your vim and vigor. You can use your fists to rub this area, the same way some that people rub their lower back when they stand up to stretch and sort of lean backward a little. This rubbing is often done before or after practices, or if you feel your energy waning. Better than a cup of joe!

Bubbling Spring

Also called Bubbling Well or Yong Chuan, this point on each foot is located in the front part of the instep near the ball of the foot. It allows you to feed your Dan Tien and Ming Men with chi from the earth. If stimulated properly, the point can help feed even more vitality up into your Dan Tien by helping to prime your Ming Men. Got that?

Stand up for a minute. Don't jiggle around or move. Just feel how your feet are placed on the floor. Many people subconsciously stand on the outside of their feet or with their weight sort of thrown back on their heels. Where is your weight placed? Are you rolling one way or the other on your feet? Planting yourself firmly (see Chapter 7 for information on T'ai Chi principles and Chapter 8 for the basics) allows your Bubbling Spring points to fully access chi from the earth and feed it up to your body's command central.

You can massage the balls of your feet with your hands to stimulate this acu-point, also. Maybe you can talk your spouse, significant other, or a good friend to do it, pleading lack of chi.

Lao Gong

If you cup your hand as if you are trying to hold water to drink, right in the center of the bottom is the Lao Gong acupoint. (Translated, you can call it the Labor or Labored Palace.) Pronounced like an exclamation of pain *(ow)* with an "l" sound in front, the Lao Gong *(gong,* rhymes with King Kong) is an energy point that I use in this book. The energy from this point is usually the easiest for someone just beginning to experiment with the flow of his or her chi. Look for a great little exercise, Feeling Your Chi, in Chapter 14.

Bai Hui

Balanced in the tippy top of your head, the Bai Hui (pronounced *by hway*) lit-erally means "hundred meetings" because many energy channels up and down your body converge in the head and mix before continuing their jour-ney. In Indian practices, the point is called the Crown Chakra.

Practicing powerfully and quietly

The essence of Qigong lies in the deep internal stillness it promotes through breath and some movement. It is a stillness that exists even when you are moving. Exercises that aren't so active are usually easier for novices to use to grasp the flow of chi. (I introduce some of these exercises in Chapter 14.) Longer forms, such as the traditional Wild Goose, string together twists, turns, bends, and reaches, and they move all around. Such forms are complicated, although experiencing them is worth the effort to seek out further instruction after you can focus on the flow of your chi. You don't want to practice Wild Goose if you must chase your chi around like a, well, wild goose.

Keeping it simple

If you try the more complicated forms too early, you'll be too busy trying to untangle your feet and arms to even remember what chi means.

In Chapters 18 and 19, I offer some ways to use Qigong alone or in combination with T'ai Chi. Take a look at these suggestions and then use your imagination to travel your own path as you weave bits of Qigong into your T'ai Chi practice.

Nurturing patience

Whether you can really pick up the essence of Qigong from a book depends on how you think and learn. Everybody can get an idea of what this practice is all about and what the movements should look and feel like. But Qigong is about finding the inner energy center and then activating it. Some people may have a great sense of what this means, and they may be able to feel the practice on their own through the movements that they find in any book, including this one. Others may crunch through some movements, wonder what it's all about, and figure it's only poppycock.

If you're intrigued but can't seem to feel the energy on your own, taking a class or workshop can work wonders. A good instructor can help you feel the energy and coax you into letting go just a bit. The energy of the class can also help you unkink your energy highway, too. If you need to experience an activity, seek your local resources by looking in your area telephone book, or start with some sources in the Appendix.

Bottom line: Try the movements and exercises in Chapter 14, 18 and 19 and get an idea of how they feel. Be patient. Even with a group or a teacher, it may take you weeks or months to begin to feel the energy flow. Qigong is not a quick fix. This practice is crock-pot cookery, not microwave magic.

Chapter 14

Meditating and Moving the Qigong Way

· ·

In This Chapter

▶ Energizing the Qigong way

▶ Standing like a tree

▶ Feeling your chi

▶ Uncovering The Eight Treasures

· ·

*W*hether you decide to take on Qigong (pronounced chee-*gung* or, as some say, chee-*gong*) as a part of your T'ai Chi practice is a personal decision based on your schedule, needs, and interests. To help decide what's best for you, take a look at Chapter 13 for more information about Qigong.

In the hands-on way, you can also thumb through this chapter and try a few basic Qigong movements. If they feel good, you may say, "Hey! I like this!" I encourage you to test it out, just for fun. Come on, humor me! Qigong's meditative ways can help you get in touch with your inner energy, which is what makes it a vital part of your T'ai Chi practice — even in tiny doses. If you look at Chapter 13, you find that Qigong's emphasis is on getting in touch with your energy flow. Tap into that, and your T'ai Chi takes 10 steps forward.

Going Forward with Qigong

So, onwards you go on your journey in Asian internal and mindful arts. This chapter is where you get to stand up and experiment.

One note before I go on: Just like with T'ai Chi, there are a million-billion (okay, maybe I'm exaggerating) teachers, styles, and types of Qigong. Over the centuries, the "recipe" was altered a bit from family to family and from generation to generation — in the same way that any chocolate chip cookie recipe can get changed from being passed around. But keep an open mind.

Some styles move more, some move less, some emphasize breathing techniques, some emphasize other aspects, some recommend more repetitions, and some less.

Although Qigong is a very gentle movement, you should consult a physician or other health care professional to make sure that they are safe for you, especially if you have any kind of orthopedic problem or if you have any neck or back injuries.

The moves that follow represent a sampling of different styles — like a Qigong appetizer. In Chapters 17, 18, and 19, I show you some ways to use not only T'ai Chi but also Qigong in short sessions as well as in combination with each other.

Nevertheless, if the concepts behind this art form intrigue you — even if my exact movements do not — press on, my friend! Take a look at the Appendix for additional resources, because there are many, many different schools and styles, some very still and some very active. Always, always continue your journey!

Standing Like a Tree

Granted, just standing without any movement can be difficult — especially for beginners. Your mind wanders off to make your to-do list while your body starts to twitch or itch. But the Standing Like a Tree forms — which aren't moving, of course — are important calming stances and powerful developers of the mind and energy flow.

Whether you want to work toward doing some standing meditations for 20 to 30 minutes, or you want to incorporate a couple of minutes at the beginning or end of a T'ai Chi routine (or before you go to bed at night), they are worth a try.

Figure 14-1 not only shows you the proper standing form but also shows you some of the possible hand positions. You don't have to do them all, but you can pick one or two that fit your mood. You can use other foot positions, too, such as the Riding a Horse stance in Chapter 8. But that's much more difficult.

I admit, it does seem odd in this fast-paced society to be asked to just stand in place. Especially since Qigong doesn't ask you to do anything physical while you're standing there — unlike Type-A behavior that applauds doing several things at the same time. If you're uncomfortable standing, try sitting at first. But be aware that the Chinese believe that you're more likely to stay quietly alert while standing. Meditations aren't naps in disguise.

The beauty of simply standing is that you feel your body and become aware of the chi and its movement. Also, you become aware of any tension in your body, and you can let your breath go to the spot and help release it. Need a reminder about chi? Take a look at Chapter 3, where I discuss chi and the basic concepts of mindful activities. If you want to find out about the various energy points or the energy channels in the body, take a look at Chapter 13.

Here are a few final tips to do your best tree-like standing:

✔ If an odd thought bounces through your mind, acknowledge it and then let it go.

✔ Keep your eyes open but relaxed, practicing the inward focus. For more information about inward focus, refer to Chapter 3 about the foundation of mind-body movement.

✔ Try playing soft music without vocals if doing so helps you focus. If you find yourself truly listening to it — not to mention tapping your toes or swaying to the rhythm — turn off the music.

✔ Start with holding the position for 2 to 3 minutes and, if you want, gradually build your time to 20 to 30 minutes.

✔ Experiment with different hand positions to see which ones feels best to you. You can hold one hand position for the entire time or change positions every few minutes.

Now it's time to stand! Try the following hand positions.

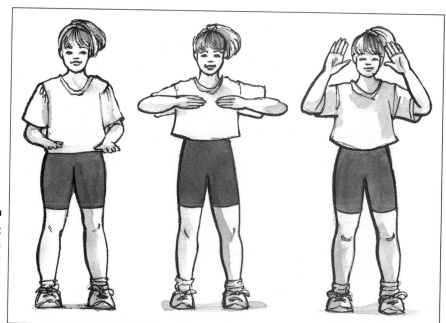

Figure 14-1:
Stand up and (don't) clap your hands like a tree.

Hang hands at side

This is the simplest position because you assume the basic standing posture with your arms at your sides. That's it. Stay in this position and follow the preceding tips for your meditation.

Place palms on table top

Hold your hands in front of your hips with the palms facing down and the elbows slightly bent. Fingers are facing forward and are spread slightly without being forced. You feel as if you have your palms resting on a hip-high table in front of you.

Embrace the tree

Hold your arms out in front of you with the elbows soft and rounded. See Chapter 8 for a reminder about T'ai Chi arms and other basics. A slight curve goes from your shoulder down to your fingertips. Imagine that you are hugging a tree very gently.

Hold arms chest high

Lift your elbows to shoulder-height beside you so your hands are at chest-height in front of you. Your palms face down, and your fingers remain a few inches apart.

Frame your face

This is the most advanced position because it takes the most endurance to hold your arms up. From the chest-height hand position, lift your hands up so your fingers are just below eyebrow-height. You kind of look like you are holding very large binoculars except your palms are turned slightly more outward and your fingers are softly extended.

Feeling your chi

Try this position sitting or standing. If you're sitting, make sure that you have good T'ai Chi Posture (see Chapter 8). Also, make sure that your feet are flat on the floor so your Bubbling Spring acupoint is fully in contact with the floor. It doesn't matter what kind of shoes, if any, you wear. If you want to find out more about the acupoints, including the Bubbling Spring, see Chapter 13.

You can even try this movement sitting in a class or in a meeting or while you are stuck standing in a grocery store line. Who knows? Maybe the energy that you generate can help you feel better — not only at that moment but all day long.

Feel your chi following these guidelines:

1. **Let your palms face each other so the distance between is from 6 inches to 1 or 2 feet.**

2. **Allow the energy emitting from each palm to connect and circulate through your body.**

   You can choose something to visualize between your palms, such as a glowing ball that you're holding, a light beam moving between your palms, or an electrical current blazing between the two.

3. **Feel a warmth in your palms, and feel it moving back and forth between them.**

4. **Try stretching your palms open and closed — as if you are pulling taffy between them — to prime your hands' energy pump.**

5. **Try slowly circling your palms as if you are rolling a large piece of dough into a ball between your palms.**

You may be surprised with the warmth that begins to emanate from your palms. Remember this feeling and apply it in other movements, too.

Microcosmic orbit

Also called Small Heavenly Circulation

This movement gets a bit esoteric, so stay with me. However, it's an awfully important concept for such a small movement. This "movement" may not actually move as you progress — at least to the casual observer.

You use this to figure out how to move your chi in its orbit through your body. (See the explanation for the microcosmic orbit in Chapter 13.) At first, you let your hands and arms take part in the circling to help move along your chi. Then you stop the movement of your hands and arms so you can try to feel the chi circulating on its own.

Truly controlling and feeling the orbit of your chi without your arms can take months. When you first experiment with this, you may want to try only Steps 1 through 4, and then add Step 5 when you're comfortable. After you feel at ease with these steps, you can move on to Step 6.

1. **Stand centered over both feet with your hands relaxed at your sides.**

2. **Inhale through the nose, feeling the breath and energy move with the breath from the base of the spine up your back to the Bai Hui acupoint in the crown of your head. As you inhale, let your hands and arms move freely and loosely upward as if tracing the circular path on the outside of your body.**

3. Exhale and feel the breath and the energy move from your crown back down the front of your body to your perineum at the base of your torso between your thighs. Let your hands and arms simultaneously mimic that path down the front as they continue their soft circle toward the front while remaining at your sides.

4. Do 9 full cycles as your orbit "warm-up."

5. After your chi is moving, forget the pattern of the breath. Just feel your chi and imagine it circling in your body on its own.

6. Drop your hands, let your body and mind take over the job, and continue the orbiting.

There are no preconceived notions about how your body reacts to Step 6. Some people may not move their bodies. Other people may sway, rise, and sink as if possessed. Just let your body move comfortably. Don't force it one way or the other.

Qigong Walking

Walking, schmalking — this movement isn't your normal heel-toe gig. This forward-moving motion is more meditation than transportation, and it certainly isn't fitness walking. So abandon the thought that this kind of walking can take the place of any real aerobic activity.

Qigong Walking is a bit like T'ai Chi Walking (see Chapter 17) because each step becomes a moment of quiet, stable meditation. Basically, it's a moving meditation similar to T'ai Chi forms but with less choreography to get wrapped up in.

When you first do this exercise, you may have to focus harder on the actual movement than the accompanying meditation. That's okay. Then, when you get the details and stability down, think about your inner peace and your energy flow.

This movement is also great balance training, which is good for anyone prone to sprained ankles or for seniors who may be prone to falls. Figure 14-2 illustrates the first and last steps.

Here are a few walking guidelines:

✔ Try to practice your Qigong Walking outdoors where you have trees, plants, animals, and green around you, if possible.

✔ Find a smooth surface so you can let go of focusing on the ground and on where your steps are going.

✔ You may find yourself more successful at Qigong Walking if you've done a few moments of standing meditation first, such as Standing Like a Tree.

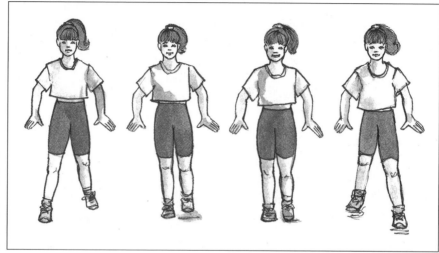

Figure 14-2:
Four out of
five Qigong
Walking
steps.

1. **Place your hands in the Table Top position (see Figure 14-1) and then float your hands to your sides as if you are propping yourself up between parallel bars to let your legs swing freely. Your fingers should face front and your hands should feel light.**

2. **Step out with your right foot, softly planting your heel first so your left foot is** *full* **(weight-bearing) and your right foot is** *empty* **(non-weight-bearing). (See Chapter 8 to get the scoop on the concepts of empty and full.)**

3. **Slowly roll through your right foot as you transfer your weight onto the right foot so the left foot becomes empty.**

4. **To transition between steps, pull the rear foot forward (in this case, the left foot) and touch the ball of the foot and toe beside your right foot. Keep it empty. This step is similar to the T'ai Chi Centering Step in Chapter 8.**

5. **Move the left foot forward and repeat the directions in Steps 2 through 4 on the opposite side.**

   You can continue this walking meditation for several minutes and then increase your time after you become more comfortable.

Your next challenge: After the forward motion is comfortable, try the movement moving backward, leading with the ball (rather than the heel) of your foot. This movement is somewhat difficult, so don't jump into it!

Take a look at the following tips for your most advantageous Qigong Walking:

✔ Stay strong and stable like an oak tree.

✔ Move slowly.

> ✔ Avoid a big thunkety-clunk when you put down your heel or toes.
>
> ✔ Relax the leg muscles when your leg becomes "empty." (See Chapter 8 for details on empty and full.)
>
> ✔ Breathe! You may be surprised how easy this part is to forget. Refer to Chapters 3 and 4 for information about how important full breaths are to gaining benefits.

The Eight Treasures

Also called The Eight Brocades, The Eight Pieces of Brocade, The Eight Silken Movements, or The Eight Sets of Embroidery

Newcomers to Qigong may practice The Eight Treasures first. That's not only because the movements are relatively simple, but also because they cover many aspects of what someone can gain from practicing Qigong. A good way to try The Eight Treasures is as a warm-up or cool-down for your T'ai Chi routine or even as your traditional exercise gambit.

You may see many names and variations of Qigong movements, but don't be taken aback. The intent, as always, is the same. Simply choose the one that best suits your needs and is most comfortable for your body. If you like The Eight Treasures but find something uncomfortable in the version that I present, take a look at the appendix and do some digging around for another version that suits you better.

All the individual movements have widely varied names, just as the title "The Eight Treasures" does. I don't give you the variations, but I pick one name for each movement. If you find this set elsewhere, you'll see that the names are similar enough that you won't be baffled.

This routine has eight movements. (Well, no kidding, Sherlock.) They are done in order and as a continuous exercise when done traditionally. (In Chapter 18, I take a less traditional route and take a few of the movements out of context for emphasis on a particular benefit. Don't be alarmed! The Qigong powers won't strike you down.)

Consider the set a moving meditation, so don't just crank them out herky-jerky like a set of calisthenics. Instead, make sure that you are inhaling and exhaling fully and deeply, using the principles for breathing (see Chapter 4 and 7). And try to maintain a smooth transition between each movement so they flow together. A transition, in this case, may only require stepping wide apart or bringing your feet together.

Do each of the movements 8 to 16 times — 8 to 10 is usually a good number, but use your judgment. Whatever number you choose, make sure that you repeat each movement the same number of times. You can't start cutting corners if you get tired, so you may want to start with fewer repetitions and see whether you have enough mental and physical endurance before you add more.

Each movement has internal and external health benefits, which I give you at the beginning of each movement.

Holding Up the Sky with Both Hands (#1)

This movement aligns and harmonizes the metabolism of the "triple burner" or "triple warmer," which is the three parts of the body (lower, middle, and upper). It teaches good balance and builds strong ankles.

1. **Start standing in good T'ai Chi Posture (see Chapter 8).**

2. **Interlace your fingers low in front of your body, keeping your palms facing down.**

3. **Slowly lift your interlaced fingers upward along your body. When they reach chest-height, rotate the palms so they face skyward.**

4. **Continue their path straight upward and slowly lift yourself onto your toes so your heels are about an inch or two off the ground. Stretch the arms and palms to the sky as if you are "holding up the sky."**

5. **Unlace the fingers and let the palms float down to your sides, keeping your heels up. When the hands reach your sides, you can drop your heels (still thinking steady balance and making no big clunks).**

6. **Repeat Steps 1 through 5 to continue the movement.**

Opening the Bow to the Left and to the Right (#2)

This stretches and strengthens the lungs as you widely open and close your arms to your sides. It strengthens the chest, shoulders, and arms. Refer to Figure 14-3. Now, if you happen to be an archer, don't be offended by the use of the word "opening" instead of "drawing" (a bow). This move isn't a Robin Hood lesson, but it's Qigong energizing.

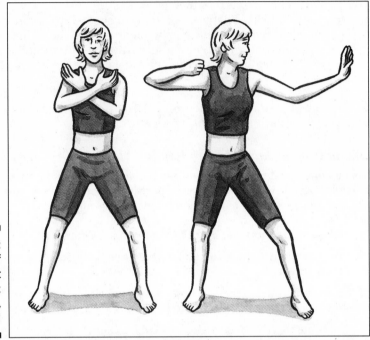

Figure 14-3:
Second of
The Eight
Treasures:
Robin Hood,
move over!

1. From your correct and balanced standing posture, take one big step to your left to assume the Riding the Horse stance (see Chapter 8).

2. Cross your left arm across your chest, palm in, so the palm is at about shoulder-height. The left fingers assume a "shooting" position, with the first finger extended; the other three fingers are curled in to the palm, and the thumb is cocked in to the palm. Your right arm crosses your chest over your left arm. The right fingers are in a loose fist. When you get the hand position down, assume the crossed-body position as you step out into the wide stance.

3. Look to the left, exhale, and uncurl your left arm to your side with the wrist cocked back as you "push" your palm to your left. Pull your right elbow back high to your side as if you are pulling the strings of a bow to shoot an arrow. Feel the stretch across the chest.

4. Push off your right foot to close it in to your left foot and return to a standing position. At the same time, pull in your left arm across your body, keeping the elbow straight and starting to relax the fingers, while your right hand simply pulls in farther across your chest.

5. Your hands are in the opposite starting position. Repeat the entire routine, stepping out to the right with the right palm pushing out, to complete one cycle.

Raising One Single Hand (#3)

This movement improves the function of the spleen and stomach to enhance digestion and immunity. It stretches the torso and breathing muscles and the upper back. Refer to Figure 14-4.

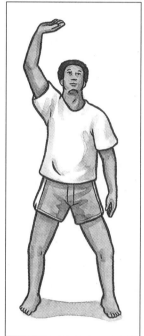

Figure 14-4:
Third of
The Eight
Treasures:
Call on me,
please!

1. **Stand with your hands palms up at about waist-height. Inhale before you begin.**

2. **Rotate the left palm out and then push it straight up above your head, as you simultaneously rotate your right palm out and down and push it down to your side. Exhale as you push up and push down.**

Be sure to keep the fingers of the downward hand pointing straightforward and keep the fingers of the upward hand pointing across your body and to the opposite side. Push strongly with your arms in opposite directions.

3. **Return your hands to the center position and repeat on the opposite side.**

Looking Behind You (#4)

This one stimulates the blood circulation in your brain, improves vision, tones the central nervous system, and gets rid of fatigue. It also prevents neck and upper-shoulder tension by stretching and releasing stress in the area, which can improve posture. Refer to Figure 14-5.

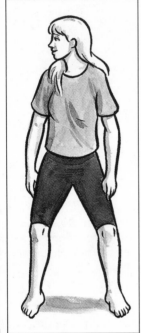

Figure 14-5: Fourth of The Eight Treasures: Is anyone following me?

1. **Stand straight with your wrists flexed slightly so your palms face down, fingers forward. Your elbows bend slightly so the hands feel as if they are floating. Inhale before you begin.**

2. **Turn your head and look over your left shoulder as far as you can without straining or pulling your torso around with you and then exhale.**

   Avoid lifting or dropping your chin as you look behind you. But let your eyes look farther behind you than your head can rotate.

3. **Repeat turning your head to the opposite side for one repetition.**

Bending Over and Wagging Head and Tail (#5)

This decreases *heart fire,* or all the things like worrying, stress, emotional anxiety, headaches, and insomnia. It also increases flexibility in your back and spine. Refer to Figure 14-6.

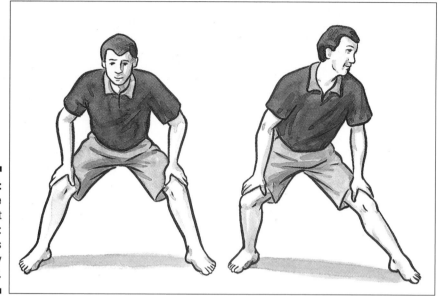

Figure 14-6:
Fifth of The Eight Treasures: Wagging is a friendly activity.

1. **Start in a Riding the Horse stance (see Chapter 8 for a description) with your hands on the top part of your thighs, thumbs pointing backward so the space between your thumb and first finger cups the thigh muscle. Keep your torso and spine straight.**

   If the wide stance is too much for you to hold, bring your feet a little closer together and gradually work on widening it.

2. **Bend forward a little from the hips (keeping the spine straight to prevent slouching). Keep the feet rooted on the floor and the toes relaxed.**

3. **Move your upper body and head toward your left thigh to start a small, controlled circling motion. Continue the circling so the torso moves down in front of you to your right thigh and then back up to the center slightly. As your torso circles to the front, your tail "wags" or makes a circling movement behind you.**

4. **Repeat the wagging and circling, starting at the right thigh first.**

5. **Stay in the Riding the Horse Stance for a few moments.**

Reaching Down to Toes (#6)

This movement empowers the kidney and brings strong chi into your upper body. It stretches the back, waist, and hamstrings. Refer to Figure 14-7.

If you have any back problems, consult with your physician before attempting the forward-hanging posture in this movement or the backward bend. Your physician can help you find a way to modify the forward-hanging movement so you support your upper back with your hands on your thighs. You can also eliminate the backward bend.

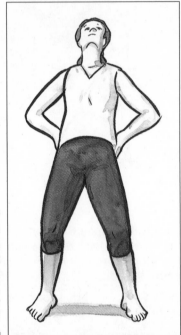

Figure 14-7: Sixth of The Eight Treasures: One, two, touch your toes!

1. **Stand with your arms at your sides. Inhale and lift your arms to your front and then upward, fingers in and palms out. Exhale and begin to circle the arms backward; then release your elbows so you can place your hands on your lower back above your buttocks.**

2. **Bend backward just a little, lifting your chest upward and using your hands in your lower back to support the weight of your upper body.**

3. **Release forward from your hips so your upper body and head starts to move forward toward the ground. At the same time, let your hands slide down the back of your buttocks and legs as far as they can go.**

4. **Release your hands and try to touch your toes.**

5. **Inhale and let your arms reach out in front of you, fingers in and palms out, as you return your upper body to an upright position. Let your arms continue to circle backward as you exhale and release your hands back to your lower back.**

6. **Repeat Steps 2 through 5 to continue the movement.**

Punching with Angry Eyes (#7)

This movement stimulates concentration, the flow of chi, the liver, and the elimination of toxins. It also builds strength in the legs, arms, and upper back.

In your modern world, perhaps letting out anger is common. You likely have so many opportunities every day to get mad, but you should actually control it. So think of being very intent with your gaze, like a focused athletic competitor who is burning a path with his or her eyes. Refer to Figure 14-8.

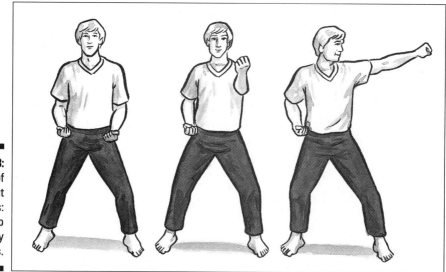

Figure 14-8:
Seventh of
The Eight
Treasures:
Fire up
those angry
eyes.

1. **Stand with your feet about 3 feet apart in a slightly modified Riding the Horse stance (see Chapter 8).**

2. **Pull both hands in, palms up, to your waist with your elbows pulled back and squeezed in. Both hands are in fists with fingers and palms up. Your hands and body are relaxed. Inhale before you begin.**

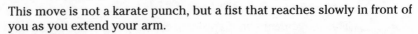

3. **Extend your left arm in front of you while rotating your arm so the fingers are down. Don't overextend or lock your elbow joint. While you extend your left arm, pull your right elbow back a little farther and squeeze tightly with both fists.**

4. **Get "angry," or intense and focused. Exhale as you press outward with your fist.**

   This move is not a karate punch, but a fist that reaches slowly in front of you as you extend your arm.

5. **Return the left arm to the starting position and relax your arms, fists, and body.**

6. **Repeat on the opposite side.**

Jolting the Back of the Body (# 8)

This movement works the adrenal glands and the kidneys to eliminate illness, and it massages the internal organs to release chi. It also strengthens the ankles and calves and stretches the spine. Refer to Figure 14-9.

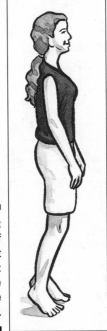

Figure 14-9: Eighth of The Eight Treasures: Caffeine isn't the only jolt.

1. **Start in an upright posture with your arms hanging at your side and palms held softly against your thighs.**

2. **Inhale and push the top of your head straight up, rising as high as you can on your toes by pushing them into the ground.**

   You can be more successful at lifting upward and staying balanced if you keep your weight forward over your toes and focus your energy on your Dan Tien. Refer to Chapter 13 if you want more information about the Dan Tien, as well as the significance of rooting yourself to the ground, which is very important if you want to stay upright!

3. **Hold for a second and then exhale and return to the starting position.**

4. **Repeat Steps 1 through 3 as many times as needed to continue the movement.**

Part V
Making the Most of Your Practice

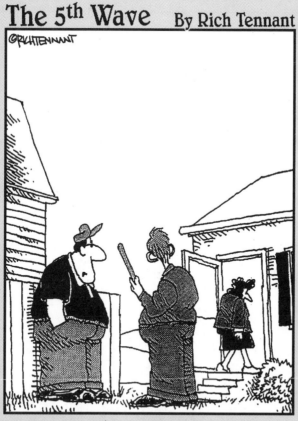

The 5th Wave   By Rich Tennant

"Sandy says she's going to repulse the monkey. I can only hope it has something to do with her T'ai Chi routine or we could be in trouble with the local zoo."

In this part . . .

Your T'ai Chi journey is now officially underway. This part is where you find out how to choose a teacher, select classes, pick reference materials (such as books or videos), or even how to go it alone with your practice. I also give you a short segment on how to start living a T'ai Chi lifestyle. But the fun isn't over yet, because now you can get moving. In this part, you also find three chapters that do nothing but show you how to put together forms — T'ai Chi and Qigong — with an array of examples that you can choose from in your practice.

Chapter 15

Practicing What I Preach

. . . .

In This Chapter

▶ Finding instructions for your T'ai Chi discovery

▶ Analyzing the ins and outs of going solo

▶ Knowing what credentials mean

▶ Selecting videos, books, or tapes

. . . .

*B*efore you start Grasping Bird's Tails, you may want to think about the best way and place are for doing all the grasping. After all, thinking through which of those fits your needs and personality, and then sorting out the best plan to bring your practice to fruition can build long-term success and more enjoyment.

In this chapter I present some ideas that will help you along the path.

Don't forget to refer to the Appendix as one primary resource for books, Web sites, instruction, conferences, associations, and other places and people that can give your practice a kick-start.

After you read this chapter and think about what's best for you, you also need to let go and just experience a little. Because one of the joys of any mindful practice such as T'ai Chi is, of course, the process. The process is the really vital part of the learning. That means that if you happen into a class somewhere, then discover you don't think you made the right choice, you haven't truly wasted a minute. You're still a step closer to your goal; you still learned not only a little T'ai Chi but also just a little bit about yourself and what you really need.

The words in this chapter about setting up your practice and finding instruction, then, represent just the first stage of your lifelong journey.

Investigating Instruction

Because you have this book, it's pretty obvious that you've got an open mind about the possibility of taking on a T'ai Chi practice on your own. Still, classes can be a great asset to learning this movement because seeing the forms demonstrated by a good teacher and experiencing the energy of a class can offer great rewards.

So, in this section I discuss the ins and outs of both going solo and searching out a class — plus related things such as deciding on a teacher — to help you move forward to grasp, repulse, part, and center the T'ai Chi way.

Going solo

You better be a truly disciplined person if your only T'ai Chi path is going to be a solo path. You should also be ready to invest in videos, other books, and occasional special workshops so you don't simply reinforce mistakes that you don't recognize. Videos will be your best asset because then you get the visual images and the flow that books (yes, even this one, I hate to say it) can't truly impart.

That's not to say you can't go solo. You can. Just have an open mind and be prepared to supplement your home practice with other education. Take a look at the next two sections for information you'll need about classes and teachers as well as about multimedia and Internet instruction and resources.

Picking your practice setting

Some activities, sports, or exercises can require you to practice in certain kinds of locations because they require particular things — mats, equipment, and so forth — that may only be available at a club or studio. T'ai Chi does not require these things, however, which is one of its beauties, especially for the solo practitioner.

Your practice setting may:

- ✔ Be any place with space to move, or at least someplace where you can move tables or a sofa out of the way. This could also be a backyard, local park, or large driveway, if the weather is comfortable for you and it's convenient.

- ✔ Be any space that can be closed off with doors or dividers so you will be free not only from distractions (kids, music, doorbells, and the like), but also from intimidation and inhibitions. This may not apply to you if you are one of those who doesn't care about others watching, or if you're a bit more advanced and are more comfortable performing the movement.

✔ Have any kind of floor, be it hardwood, tile, carpet, or wood, or other surface such as concrete, or grass — so long as your feet and legs are comfortable as you move.

That's it! You don't even need music, which frees you from needing a particular sound system, boom box, and so forth.

I once took a class from a man who held classes in the back courtyard of a community center. Some of the people in the group were on grass, some were on concrete, and some were on both as they moved. People came and went from the community center, driving in and out of the back parking lot behind us and walking in and out of the back door in front of us. Once we got going on our T'ai Chi, however, these potential distractions didn't really matter. The classes that my collaborator Manny took were usually held in a local park.

A couple of additional needs concern how you feel about your chosen space:

✔ **The space needs to feel safe.** This can mean different things to different people. When you go to your space, however, you need to feel okay about doing what you do at whatever level of proficiency you do it. If you think someone is peeking at you, which makes you uneasy, you won't be as diligent about your practice.

✔ **The energy in the space needs to feel positive.** This requirement is pretty hard to really explain because it's all about a gut feeling and listening to your heart and soul. I'm sure you've been places where you were uneasy for some reason or you felt antsy, uncomfortable, or tense. In other places, however, you may feel at ease, filled with energy, peaceful, and calm. Make sure your T'ai Chi place falls into the latter category.

Settling on your environment

The objects around you in your space represent another matter entirely. Because of T'ai Chi's reliance on chi (see Chapter 3 for more on that), being outside is actually ideal. Why? The living trees, green grass, soulful earth, and shifting skies can help you tap into your own chi better because they have so much to offer.

If you can't be outside, though, try to have an indoor setting that brings the outdoors in. Here are a few suggestions for doing just that:

✔ Have plants in the room where you practice. Make sure they are healthy plants so their chi is also healthy.

✔ Large windows that let in dawn's light, dusk's setting sun, or the blue sky can help create a more pleasant area.

✔ Play tapes of peaceful nature sounds, such as water or birds, softly in the background if it helps you. Other types of music, however, can be distracting. (Some purists avoid music whatsoever.)

✔ Think about investing in one of those indoor burbling fountains so you can hear real water near you.

✔ Light candles or incense, if you like that touch. Some people don't like these things, and they're not as common in T'ai Chi classes as they are in other types of mindful exercise.

Assembling your accessories

Compared to other mind-body methods — such as Yoga or Pilates — that need specific clothes, particular equipment, or certain accessories, T'ai Chi is pretty simple, which makes it even more accessible and affordable.

The first thing you need is a space and an appropriate environment, as I describe in the preceding sections. As long as you have your space, you can actually just start into your forms and stances and be a happy T'ai Chi camper.

The other thing that can make you an even happier camper, however, is your clothes. No, you don't need any special outfits — unless you go to certain studios that require particular uniforms. But you're still going solo here, so all you need is something that's comfortable and lets you move without binding, pinching, or bulking up in all the wrong places.

To outfit yourself more comfortably try:

✔ **Bottoms:** Loose sweatpants or drawstring pants such as those used in some Yoga practices work well. Even tights work because they move with you like a second skin.

✔ **Tops:** Loose tops, such as t-shirts or sweatshirts, are great. If a woman is comfortable with it, she can just put on a sport bra and leave it at that. If it's hot, a man can certainly — if he's practicing on his own at least — go shirtless.

✔ **Footwear:** There are several schools of thought on footwear:

Some beginners just wear athletic shoes, such as walking or running shoes. These types may work especially well if you are on cement, wood, or another hard surface.

You can also choose soft and thin slipper-like shoes because they offer you a better feel for the ground and force you to rely only on yourself for balance, not your shoes. You may find a slip-on Asian slipper in some import stores that works well. They have thin rubber soles.

You can also go barefoot, which works especially well if you're on carpet or grass. Going barefoot gives you a great feel for nature and its part in your practice. Make sure that there is no chance to stumble on broken glass or other hazards, however, especially if you are in a public park.

Aside from these items, you will probably want to have a towel handy if the weather is hot. And whether it's hot or not, you'll want to have a bottle of water handy to sip on before or after your forms.

That's all the accessories that you need. Now isn't T'ai Chi just so simple?

Timing it best

I get asked all the time about when is the best time to exercise. My typical answer is, "Any time that you'll do it." The same applies to T'ai Chi. Pick the time that best fits your schedule and your life's demands, and do it then. Convenience is a huge factor in the lives of busy people, so don't ignore its import.

There are, of course, two truly ideal times. Which one is better for you, however, depends on your needs:

- ✔ **Dawn:** Something about the rising sun and its energy changing from softer yin to more energetic yang (for more on that see Chapter 3) can make a practice at this time of day a true energizer. It's a good way to feel balanced and calm as you set out for the day ahead.

- ✔ **Twilight:** Just like with the changing light and energies at dawn, the opposite occurs at sunset. The sun sinks and the energy changes from the more aggressive yang to a gentler yin. A practice at this time of day will set you up for a calmer evening, perhaps even settling you after a busy day.

Pick the time you'll do it, but also try to experience both of these times.

Setting up your structure

Deciding what to practice and for how long is a very personal decision. What you choose can depend on:

- ✔ Your reasons for practicing.
- ✔ Your preferences in movement.
- ✔ How long you can devote to your practice sessions.

Manny, my collaborator, didn't fiddle-faddle around. As a beginner, he spent between 90 minutes to 2 hours each of 4 to 5 days a week on his own, as well as attending class for 3–4 hours one weekend morning. No, no, don't freak out or close the book and tuck it up on a high shelf because you don't have that kind of time. Really, you don't have to commit so much time. That's just one example of one end of the spectrum.

No matter how much time you spend each day or each week, however, fitting in a few parts can help you advance more quickly. Simply adjust the time you spend on each part. For example, if you have 30 minutes, spend 5–10 minutes on each component. If you have 90 minutes, you can spend 20 minutes or more on each, give or take, based on your emphasis.

Here are the basic practice session components to include, in order:

1. **Warm-up exercises:** Do something that stimulates your circulation, and then follow that with some stretching and loosening movements. See Chapter 8 for suggestions. *Time allotment:* About 25 percent of the session.

2. **Stance training and meditation:** You can either do these separately or together. Because you can meditate while in stances, however, doing them together makes sense. Meditating while in T'ai Chi stances also helps you to develop greater relaxation and to build up chi and inner strength much better than just sitting and meditating. *Time allotment:* About 25 percent of the session.

3. **Form training:** This is why you bought your ticket, so to speak — to learn the forms, be it the Yang Short or Long or some other. So now that you've got a good chunk of time to devote to form training, personal learning preferences kick in again. You can do a Yang form all the way, and then go back and practice a few sequences in it repetitively, then do it all together again. Or you can go over a few forms that have caused you problems and then do it all together. Or you may want to do just 2–3 forms in the sequence a few times through — especially if you have limited time. After you get more proficient, you'll be able to do several entire repetitions of a Yang form. What you choose will depend a little on not only how much time you have, but also on your goals for the session. *Time allotment:* About 50 percent of the session.

4. **Qigong finale:** Sometimes finishing up with a little bit of Qigong can leave you refreshed and ready to go, but this also depends on time, experience, and desire. *Time allotment:* Depends on how much time you have, and if you decide to add Qigong to your practice. (For information about what Qigong is and how it complements a practice, see Chapter 13.)

Finding a teacher or class

It would be fine flattery to me if you thought this book was all you needed for a complete T'ai Chi practice. On the other hand, if you thought this book was all you needed, I might actually be disappointed. My goal for this book is that it serves as an introductory guide or a refresher reference, because watching or listening to a live person and experiencing group dynamics can take your T'ai Chi practice up to an entirely new level.

Starting the search

You have several avenues to follow to track down a local place to go for classes or someone in your area to take lessons from, including:

- ✔ **Local health and community centers:** If you belong to a health club or gym, you may find a class right under your nose. Many fitness centers are mixing mind-body classes, including the likes of T'ai Chi and Qigong, with traditional offerings these days. Other places that are addressing T'ai Chi include community centers, adult education schools, and senior centers. I once found a free T'ai Chi class at a senior center at which all ages were welcome. It was beautifully taught in the garden behind the building, no less.

- ✔ **Inquiries with those you know or where you shop:** Ask around. Some of your friends may be taking classes and want to share their finds with you! Try asking at health food or alternative stores, or read their bulletin boards. So-called "New Age" shops (the types that sell candles and incense) often have connections to these kinds of classes, or at least can refer you.

- ✔ **Let your fingers do the walking:** Try the phone book (print or electronic version). The trick to finding T'ai Chi classes is figuring out where to look in your local phone book. The listing may be under Wellness, Fitness, Karate, Martial Arts, Mind-Body, or something else. You may also find that the names of centers can be misleading. For example, an Aikido studio (combat kinda stuff) may actually have T'ai Chi classes — or know where someone does. Don't hesitate to call and ask.

- ✔ **Referrals from national associations:** Contact a national T'ai Chi organization or association (either by phone or on the Web). Many maintain lists of teachers that you can research by area. Even if the group doesn't list someone in your area, ask further. The number of teachers is changing so quickly that groups often can't update printed or electronic lists fast enough. The Appendix in this book may help you get started.

- ✔ **Recommendations from area teachers:** If you find a teacher or class, but the location is a bit too far from you, ask that teacher if he or she knows another class or teacher located closer to you. Each method tends to have a network, and teachers know who is where and doing what. And because it's not truly competition if you're 30 miles away, T'ai Chi colleagues will usually gladly refer you.

- ✔ **Internet searches:** I get into other Internet resources later in this chapter, but you'll be surprised at how even the most local teacher or smallest of studios has a Web site containing at least contact information. Granted, such small sites may be woefully out-of-date, but they can get you started. And in fact they could be even better than larger ones because they are lovingly nutured by the teacher. Input your area of interest — and your city or metropolitan area to narrow the search — and see what comes up.

Recognizing a quality instructor

T'ai Chi instructors differ from the normal instructor that you may seek, be it movement or academic. For example, when it comes to fitness instructors, there are enough certifications and degrees out there to choke a horse, so seeing lists of those behind an instructor's or trainer's name can help in making a choice. When it comes to university professors, degrees and experience to some part are required, so that makes choosing an instructor much simpler too.

But what about internal martial arts such as T'ai Chi and Qigong? The choices can be baffling, especially to the uninitiated novice. I won't candy-coat that one.

You see, T'ai Chi is a method that is handed down through the ages and steeped in tradition, not certificates. Neither the United States nor most other countries maintain restrictions on who can teach T'ai Chi. T'ai Chi instructors don't have to have any mandatory credentials or degrees in the United States either. (There are, however, T'ai Chi teaching certifications in China that are considered quite good, although not all are good.)

So, a teacher you stumble across in the West may either be really good or may be someone who took an eight-week class and has now convinced him- or herself that he or she is ready to lead. This person may even go so far as to call him- or herself a master. Certifications do exist in the West, but no one controls what these programs teach, if they are the greatest thing since sliced bread (and some are), or if they are not better than a mail-order sweepstakes.

So there's the puzzle, leaving you the novice kind of stabbing around in the dark, hoping for a good recommendation or simple good luck. To help you along in your search for a qualified instructor — an important part of a program — take a look at these tips:

✔ **Observe and think:** If there is a studio or club with classes nearby that interest you, ask to observe a lesson taught by the teacher that would be instructing you. Watching shouldn't be an issue for the club. If it is, that's a big red warning flag. On the other hand, some reputable places will invite you to take a class for free before signing up. That's the sign of a confident instructor or studio!

When you observe the class, you should come with a few questions in mind. For example, does the style feel comfortable to you? Does the teacher communicate enough to fit your style? Does the teacher communicate too much? Do the students seem to enjoy themselves and socialize before or after, even helping each other? Is the teacher available to answer questions? Does he or she give the kind of instruction that would fit your needs? Does he or she also look smooth and confident in their forms? Does the class start and finish on time, if that's important to you? Imagine yourself in the class and how you would feel as a participant.

It may not be the sign of a bad teacher if you don't like the class. Maybe that instructor's style just doesn't fit you. After the lesson, tell the teacher about your needs and perhaps he or she can suggest other classes.

✔ **Communicate and question:** Talk to an instructor about his or her background. Make sure that the instructor isn't one of those eight-week specials who thinks that he or she knows it all. Find out how long he or she has studied, where he or she studied, and under which master or at what club. Some experts believe a teacher should have at least five years of study under their belt before embarking on teaching. Ask simple questions about T'ai Chi theory or history. A good instructor should be versed enough to answer these questions.

✔ **Listen and ask:** Ask around at the places suggested in the previous section about where to find classes. Word gets around about classes and teachers that people like, even among non-participants. So, ask.

✔ **Sign up and network:** Taking a short course at an adult or community center can be an inexpensive way to get an introduction without a huge investment. These programs often run only 4–6 weeks, so even if the instructor isn't your ideal, you'll learn a few things and be able to ask around among students about other places to go. After you connect with the T'ai Chi network, finding other resources will be easier.

Typifying a T'ai Chi class

Before you actually step into a class, knowing what to expect can be comforting. I can't give you an exact outline, of course, because every teacher and style is a bit different. How the class flows and what is done will also depend on the class's goal: Is it for health? Is it to train for combat with accomplished students of other martial arts forms? Is it for seniors more interested in balance training? Is it teaching the long or short form, Push Hands, or weapons, Chen or Yang form? (Take a look at Chapter 5 and 6 to find out more about those things.)

No matter what the goal, however, a good class will:

✔ Include some kind of warm-up, be it different movements or slower T'ai Chi or even Qigong.

✔ Incorporate some "stance training" (see Chapter 14 to read about Qigong stances, as well as Chapter 8 to read about basic T'ai Chi stances) because getting a good physical foundation is key to good chi flow and better T'ai Chi.

✔ Offer some meditation, be it short or long, as a part of stances or separately. Mediation may not be a huge aspect, depending on the goal or the teacher, but it should be introduced and done at least occasionally.

- Instruct forms, which is of course the meat of the class. See Chapters 9–11 for T'ai Chi forms.

- Break down forms. You'll work on the specific parts of one or more forms — isolating movements to perfect them — then do them all together again.

There are other expectations, of course, that have nothing to do with the forms or stances you're learning. A class should also:

- Be orderly. You have a right to expect, as a paying student, that an instructor will keep control of the students, avoid unruly behavior, and offer organized, staged learning.

- Flow seamlessly between segments.

- Be challenging. That could mean that the class is difficult, both mentally and physically. For example, a lot of stance training is not easy on leg and hip muscles, although a good teacher will know how to show students to modify instruction for their level and needs.

- Accommodate many levels, which is particularly true if a class is ongoing, with new people coming and going and regulars just plugging along. If you feel overloaded, talk to the instructor.

Merging Martial Arts with Modern Multimedia

These days you can find a wealth of information on video, from tapes, in other books, and on the Internet. Those are all valid places to seek out your instructor, at least in part.

Selecting stars of the video screen

Choosing videos may be more difficult than screening for an instructor. You usually can't observe a video once for free like you can a class, and there is no governing body that approves the production of a video.

I got one video from a leading source that, in terms of production quality, was the stuff from which nightmares are made. A man stood in his studio, back to a dirty wall, shadows in all the wrong places, and talked through his movements. He made mistakes, misspoke, was shot from bad angles, and sometimes kept talking when he turned his back to the camera — but the camera kept rolling. Note I say, in "production quality" it was poor; the instruction itself was pretty decent — if you weren't too busy being distracted by people scurrying in front of the lens.

Shaping up to get moving?

Do you have to be in shape to do T'ai Chi? Not really, because it is very gentle and great for beginners. Having some small level of fitness can help you progress much faster, however. If your muscles ache for several days after T'ai Chi — either on your own, in a class, or with a video — you are probably doing too much. Like any form of exercise, T'ai Chi should not hurt. It should be challenging, yes, but it shouldn't hurt. Good teachers will be able to help you find stance modifications to help accommodate your level. That includes instructors on videos and in books. Notice in Chapters 8–12 that I give a lot of variations and modifications for different levels.

If you practice T'ai Chi on your own, remember: An "ouch" pain that lingers more than a couple of days is one pain too much, and you should consider seeing a doctor. A muscle ache — from a complaining muscle that is shrieking about doing new things — may be okay, but it shouldn't be so bad that it limits your regular daily activities. If you do ache a little, take a day off, try putting some ice on the ache, and do some very easy stretching. If that doesn't help, see a physician

Here are a few tips for choosing a T'ai Chi video:

- ✔ Look for legitimate video sources, not only for mind-body arts but also for exercise videos (some of those companies now carry the non-traditional alongside the traditional because of increased popularity). You'll find some of these sources in the Appendix.

- ✔ Read the package cover — or catalog description — to see what kind of credentials the instructor has.

- ✔ Look for mention on covers or in catalogs not only of different camera angles but also of repetitions to help you really understand a movement.

- ✔ Try to choose something where movements are broken down into tiny pieces so you can better assimilate the forms.

- ✔ Check whether the catalog or store has a "satisfaction guaranteed" warranty, so if you watch it and discover that it is terrible, you can get a refund or at least an exchange.

- ✔ Be ready to take risks. These videos can be like grab bags! You never know if you're going to get the prize or the gag.

Reading all about it

Where to start in knowing which tome is good and which is a disaster? These tips will help:

- If you take a class, ask the teacher for recommendations for reading material. Even if you don't take a class, you can call a local club and ask for recommendations.

- If you choose to go to a bookstore, don't pick out the biggest or flashiest book you see. Decide what you really need (more explanation? more pictures? more definitions? detailed instructions?) and look specifically for that feature in a book. And, as with videos, read the author's credentials.

- If you do your shopping on the Internet, look for a store that gives you detailed descriptions, including numbers of illustrations, number of pages, and author credentials. This information will help you make a more educated choice.

The bottom line is read — read a lot. It will always help your T'ai Chi and your understanding of T'ai Chi.

However, you will find two problems with all T'ai Chi books (and, sigh, this one is not an exception, although it is *meant* to be a reference, of course):

- T'ai Chi flows without breaks with your arms, hands, feet, legs, hips and everything moving at the same time. A book — because of the mechanics of the written word — becomes segmented, leaving you to imagine the flow.

- T'ai Chi is three-dimensional; a book's pages are flat. Some people won't be able to translate the lack of dimensions on the page to real life.

Once again, see the Appendix to help you get started on filling out your library. And do consider it a reference library and not the only place you'll get instruction.

Navigating the Internet

The Internet has become an invaluable source for researching just about any topic, internal and mindful Asian arts included. Without getting into an entire lesson on how to search the Web, here are a few tips for searching the Internet for T'ai Chi information:

- Start your search by entering the name of the art you want more information about into your favorite search engine, such as Google or Yahoo!. You will get back sites to peruse. I promise.

✔ Experiment with different spellings of T'ai Chi and Qigong. Spellings, spaces, and placements of apostrophes can confuse a search engine. Also, if certain non-English words can be spelled several ways, most engines only know one spelling. For example, Qigong can also be spelled Chi Kung or Qi Gong, but may have been entered with only one of those spellings into the search engine's database and is tagged with only one of those names on the site itself. T'ai Chi can be known by its full name, T'ai Chi Chuan, or the Chinese spelling, Taijiquan. Look for alternatives in the spelling of T'ai Chi in Chapter 6, and in spelling Qigong in Chapter 13.

You can find all kinds of information on the Internet, some less formal or polished than others, but often still worth taking a look at. The Appendix will get you started.

Chapter 16

Living a T'ai Chi Lifestyle Every Day

. . . .

In This Chapter

▶ Timing your T'ai Chi practice

▶ Living the T'ai Chi life

▶ Making your body fit for T'ai Chi

. . . .

Taking on T'ai Chi or other internal martial arts is a bit different than learning, say, to sew or to swing a baseball bat. The principles aren't really something that you just practice dutifully for an hour in class, and then forget about until the next session. These principles (as I explain in Chapter 7) become a part of your blood, sweat, soul, and psyche if you truly attempt to develop a full practice.

Learning the forms is all well and good; the movements may feel good and you may feel superficially and physically stronger or more flexible. But as you learn to breathe, develop your chi, root yourself, and all those other key parts to developing good forms (discussed in Chapters 3,4, and 7), you find an amazing thing: The forms are just a path to doing and to learning all of those things I just mention. The forms are just the vehicle to get you farther along your journey — a journey that can transform your life and thoughts. These forms are only the physical expression of what is happening inside of you.

In this chapter, I take you a short step beyond the 1-2-3 how-to of forms and introduce you to — actually really only begin to skim the surface of — how the principles and concepts can help you all day every day so you can truly live your T'ai Chi. Granted, some of that introduction also comes by describing short moments where you can do some physical practice of some small aspect of T'ai Chi. As always, however, this is more about making it a part of your blood and life, rather than just perfecting your forms.

Making Changes through T'ai Chi

While you're so dutifully discovering how to Repulse the Monkey, Grasp the Bird's Tail, or develop a dandy Bow Stance (Chapters 8 through 11 explore all of those forms), something else is taking place: You also learn, for example, about the power of softness, the peace of strength, and the stillness that you can reap by using and appreciating opposites taught by the principles of yin and yang. (Chapter 3 presents an introduction to yin and yang.)

Look closely at the order of presentation, even in this book. Note that the mindful foundation of a practice as well as the principles of T'ai Chi come many pages before you get to do the forms themselves.

Actually, discovering the underlying principles of T'ai Chi and how they relate to your life can be a very personal journey because everybody's needs are different. Take what you want. Leave the rest. Then step out and explore on your own to find out where you may want to add a little T'ai Chi to your life, be it practically speaking (the next section) or philosophically speaking (right after that).

Making T'ai Chi Part of Your Day

In this section, I don't tell you when and where to do what and how. Chapters 17–19, on the other hand, make lots of specific suggestions about the kinds of forms, movements, and short combinations that you can do for a few minutes of practice now and then. This section merely presents a list of ideas to get your brain bustling on its own about how and when you can to find a few minutes for real practice, but also how to use time while doing something else to apply a movement or other physical concept.

Timing your ticket

You may want to break out of your normal mode of adding movement to your day when it comes to T'ai Chi. It's a little different than exercise where you just slot in your 30–60 minutes a few times a week. Here are a few times to consider (or reconsider):

- **Watching the sunrise:** There is something magical about watching the sun rise as warm orange and red light wash over you and your surroundings, painting everything in preparation for the day and prompting a wake-up to people still at rest. Sunrise has a stillness — even in the heart of most cities — that can create an oasis in a normally frenzied day. *Choosing* to get up early makes all the difference in how you feel about getting up early. So plan enough sleep, and then try getting up with the rooster's crow so that you can get in a few forms.

- **Minding the midmorning:** Sometimes as midmorning hits, your speed picks up as you race to lunch meetings, to home from school projects, to daycare to pick up the kids, or to another class. This time may be awkward for practicing some true T'ai Chi forms because you're in the middle of a period of daily hustle and bustle. That hustle-bustle activity, however, may be even more reason to take a moment. No matter where you are, you can find a secluded bench, an empty corner office, a spot behind a building that no one frequents, or even an empty stairwell. Instead of running for a cup of coffee, do some short meditations or less-active forms. Doing so can re-energize you for an upcoming meeting or the rest of the morning's flurry.

✔ **Doing a nooner:** Sometimes when noon rolls around, you hurry off to lunch and eat on the run, or grab a bite in the car or at your desk. Hey, take that time for yourself away from the daily routine. You will always return more refreshed than if you just drove to the local burger joint, ate, and returned to work. This time may be good for you to actually do longer forms or meditations, take in a class, or to pop in a video to follow, depending on where you are.

✔ **Mixing it up midafternoon:** Most people enter a slump period around midafternoon. Researchers even found that your body slows down about seven to eight hours after you get up. For many of us, this slump time falls between about 1 and 4 p.m. — just when a large mocha sounds appealing as a pick-me-up. Oh wait, stop. Forget the large mocha. Go for 5 to 10 minutes of easy stances instead to get your blood flowing and keep your mind alert.

✔ **Taking care of the sunset (or early evening):** Ah, another beautiful and normally peaceful time of day, especially in the late spring, summer, and early fall when the days last a bit longer. (In the dead of winter, however, sunset may come too early to truly enjoy it because it may fall practically at midafternoon! In that case, refer to the preceding bullet item.) In contrast to sunrise when you energize yourself for the day, at sunset, or in the early evening, you want to find peace with your day and slow down your pace.

✔ **Tucking in before bedtime:** Perhaps bedtime is the first time you can find for yourself during the day. Fine, just avoid what many people commonly do: Rush, rush, rush all day until bedtime comes, and then collapse into the sheets only to start the rush-rush schedule as soon as the sun rises the next day. Find a few moments to slow down before you head for zzzzzzs.

I give you some tips about creating a personal sanctuary for quiet time later in this chapter. The next three chapters (17–19) give you some sample ideas about short forms and mini-combos to help you map out your own practice. So, start thinking about what time of day you prefer and what exercises fit best into your schedule.

Plotting quick T'ai Chi escapes

In the preceding section, I point out all the large sections of your day in which you can practice T'ai Chi. How about I just toss out a few other times and places where you can squeeze in an itty-bitty T'ai Chi moment? The following situations can help you gather your own thoughts and ideas about what may work for you in your life:

- ✔ **Approaching a red traffic light:** Oh don't you just hate to see a traffic light turn yellow and then red as you approach? Don't get mad at an inanimate object by cursing and pounding on the steering wheel (and raising your blood pressure in the process). Instead, take the opportunity to breathe mindfully and conquer your haste. What good does it do to sit there and get all steamed up? None. You can't change anything. Instead, breathe and use those 60 seconds to release some tension. This applies to all those other hurry-up-and-wait things in life, too such as traffic jams, post office lines, busy restaurants . . . .

- ✔ **Dealing with someone aggravating at work (or elsewhere):** Look at that person as an ally in your efforts to develop tolerance and inner peace. Again, what good does it do you to get all keyed up about how someone else is acting? Let it roll off your shoulders and rise above it all. Use the moment to connect to your microcosmic orbit (see Chapters 13 and 14 about Qigong for information on that).

- ✔ **Holding, carrying, gripping, or typing:** When doing any sort of activity, such as driving or writing, how many times do you use more oomph than you need to? (I for one tend to pound the keyboard when I type, which is useless and definitely not very calming.) Practice using just enough muscle power to complete your activity. Take a few moments now and then during the day to take a little inventory while you hold the phone, write, type (that one's for me), or even hang onto your fork or cup for dear life. Catch the tension, release it, feed positive chi into the area, and feel more balanced.

- ✔ **Opening a heavy door:** This sounds like a funny time to practice T'ai Chi, but the principles of rooting and sinking (see Chapter 7) all come into play here. Rather than trying to muscle that dang door open with your arms, bend your knees, sink your body weight lower, and push or pull it open with your entire body moving as a unit. This allows you to practice sinking, moving your whole body in one piece, and using only the right muscles with just the right amount of force. It's pretty cool what you can do just by opening a door, huh?

- ✔ **Standing in line:** Whether you're at the grocery store, bank, or Department of Motor Vehicles, lines probably make you feel as if your life is standing still when you have a zillion things to do, right? You might sidle up close to the person in front of you as if pushing him or her forward (as if that'll help?); tap your toes (you think you're entertaining the other folks in line?); or speak curtly to the person behind you (what did that poor soul do?). In any case, you definitely are not working on the principles of T'ai Chi, including stillness and balance. You can take these moments as a gift of time to practice your T'ai Chi Posture, refine your Centering Step, tap into your microcosmic orbit, or just connect with your chi and the earth. This practice doesn't have to be dramatic, or even noticeable to the people around you. (You don't want them calling the cops on you.)

Rather than stress out over where you want to be or what you'd rather be doing, let yourself be fully present in the moment. Impatience stems from an inability to be present to what is going on in your life right now, and T'ai Chi is specifically about the process, not the goal or destination. In T'ai Chi, you never do really get there; rather you are always on your way there, learning and growing constantly as you go.

Nevertheless, a lot of people live their lives in a hurry to be someplace other than where they actually are. You miss a lot of what life has to offer when you are white-knuckling your way down the highway intent on a destination rather than enjoying the process of getting there.

Manny, my collaborator, offers this wise old Buddhist saying: "Don't let others walk in your clean mind with their dirty feet."

And that, my friend, leads me directly into the next section about simply using the principles in your daily life.

Living Your T'ai Chi Principles

You don't have to munch on mung beans and tofu to embrace T'ai Chi and its principles as a part of your life, day-in and day-out. Following a T'ai Chi path means just looking at, experiencing, and reacting to things a little differently.

T'ai Chi provides a lifelong learning experience that can color, shape, and alter every aspect of your life. It provides a means for changing your life physically, mentally, emotionally, and even spiritually. Some people are content to simply walk along the T'ai Chi path as a means to improve health or reduce stress, which is no problem and is a fine reason to follow the path. Others, however, embark upon the journey as an entirely new way of life. Both paths are valid. Even one that is halfway between the two is valid.

There are umpteen paths for you to follow in life. It is up to you to discover for yourself whether a path has the heart you seek or need.

Your T'ai Chi practice doesn't really stop then when you close this book and move on to your chores. In this section, I give you some ways to take the principles — and the wisdom you have gathered or will gather through them — for the ride as you cruise through your day.

Unplugging from stress

In addition to T'ai Chi, Manny (my collaborator) also teaches stress management classes at the hospital. His approach, due to his T'ai Chi training, differs slightly from that of some of his peers. Rather than emphasizing techniques that require a retreat to a quiet place for meditation or relaxation exercises, Manny strives instead to get people to examine and to change their attitudes, outlooks, and perceptions so that they prevent stress from ever accumulating to harmful levels. His approach is like teaching someone to fish instead of giving them a fish. Incorporating this technique can carry someone through all kinds of scenarios and places. Those changes are all related to T'ai Chi principles, such as breathing, connecting to your chi, rooting yourself, using only the muscles and power needed, and not freaking out over things you can't change. Letting go to get hold, so to speak.

Have you ever seen or met someone who just seems to float along, being effective in life, but never really being ruffled by tempests in teapots? That's you if you embrace these principles. Just as a turtle carries his home with him wherever he goes, you can carry you own little cocoon of serenity with you wherever you go.

Concentrating on breathing

In all situations, breathe. Train yourself to be aware of your breath. You may be surprised at how often you catch yourself holding your breath. Really. Especially if you're writing at a computer on a project deadline! It takes practice, but remind yourself just to check in with your body and see what it's up to, including breathing.

If you're in a conversation, debate, discussion, or even an argument with someone, take a moment to breathe before you respond. Focusing on slowing your breath can help slow your pulse and blood pressure. (See Chapter 2 for more on the physical benefits of mind-body exercise, as well as Chapter 4 for how breathing helps build mindful benefits.)

Taking a peek inside

Think about how and why you feel and react the way you do in certain situations or to certain people. Is it really something about yourself or your own frustration that you take out on the other person? Let yourself feel all during the day, in everything that you do, by looking inward in short meditative moments.

Observing the goings-on around you

Observe both yourself and others in daily interactions. Do remember, however, that T'ai Chi is all about being nonjudgmental, so just observe. Observation doesn't mean thinking, "Oh, what I just said was so stupid," or "How could she ever have worn those ugly shoes?" Observation just means noting things around you and how they affect you, then acknowledging that reaction or affect. After some time practicing these methods, you find more calm and peace day-to-day.

Responding to the behavior of others

Everyone has to deal with an inconsiderate person at work or while shopping, at least once in a while. Rather than responding in kind, maintain your courtesy and continue to treat difficult people as you wish they were treating you. When you allow the attitudes and behaviors of others to determine your responses, you give them an awful lot of power. And you give them even more power if you can't let go of some exchange, but rather continue to dwell on it or the person after the fact.

My mom and dad used to tell me to "kill them with kindness" if someone was a pain in the you-know-what, and I have continued to carry that lesson through life.

So let go, be nice, and go with the flow.

Going with your gut

If you don't believe, you probably won't ever plug into your chi. If you don't trust, you may never be able to let go enough to find the strength in stillness.

Trust and believe in trusting and believing!

Taking five

No time for T'ai Chi breaks, you say? I don't swallow that excuse. Everybody — and I do mean everybody — can find at least five minutes in the day for him- or herself. Try the little exercise where you write down every little thing you do from the time you get up until the time you go to bed. Everything. For example: brushing teeth, 2 minutes; reading the newspaper, 15 minutes; looking for car keys, 4 minutes; and so forth. After you figure out where all your time is going, you can easily figure out where to find those five minutes for your breathing, stance, or centering practice.

Find five. Make that your motto. At least five. After you find five, then begin the search for ten.

Taking Care of Your Body

Much of this book talks about your mind, your mind's effect on your body, and how you can adjust your movements to suit your body's needs. But what about what you put *in* your body as fuel? Or how you sit? How you stand? If you get enough rest?

If you treat yourself poorly all the time except when you're in class or practicing forms or stances, you also won't fully benefit from the journey. No, this book isn't about self-care, nutrition, exercise, and other related things. For that you can find tomes in the library or bookshelves. I just take a very brief look at a few areas that are important to embracing T'ai Chi as a lifestyle.

Creating a sanctuary

Finding a quiet place — a T'ai Chi sanctuary if you will — where you can feel safe to "go away" into your routine for 10, 20, or 30 minutes can be key to finding your practice time. Follow these guidelines to establish the ultimate T'ai Chi retreat:

✔ **Find a place where you can focus.** Focusing on yourself is hard enough without having a place to call your own. When you try to do T'ai Chi, you don't want to look at a cluttered desk, the kids' toys, the piles of dishes, the heaps of laundry, or the great balls o' dust in the corners.

✔ **Add items that help you forget distractions.** Room dividers or screens can help you block out the family, the mess, or the chores that you need to do. (And these dividers can be a really attractive part of your decor,

too.) Candles can also help set the stage or add a pleasant aroma to the area, if you like. A statue or a picture can help you feel as if you're really on a true retreat. Even putting on particular clothes can help put you in the mood.

✔ **Preserve your sanctuary.** Even if this space can't be permanent, look around for a corner and mentally claim it. You can then keep your "sanctuary supplies" in a drawer, on a closet shelf, or folded up under the bed. When you're ready for your mind-body retreat, just pull out the dividers, candles, and clothes, and set yourself up in a flash.

✔ **Know when to let go of your sanctuary.** Be able to take moments without relying on the physical nature of a particular spot, such as your sanctuary.

If you take care of your body (and mind!), they'll take care of you.

Eating smart

If you eat healthfully, you usually feel good and are able to focus. Eating smart means eating a diet with low fat, high fiber, moderate protein (vegetarian if you prefer but it's not mandatory), whole sources of carbohydrates, and plenty of fruits and vegetables. Take a look at menus in many Asian restaurants for an idea of the balance and proportions that work pretty well. Ever wonder why real Chinese dishes have so many vegetables and balance it all with rice? Because in most cases, they follow the kind of healthful diet that I describe — if they follow traditional meals.

Research shows that most people know what they *should* eat, but don't follow the program. Doing so takes a bit of effort sometimes. If you need a little hand (and who doesn't?), try visiting buying a simple book on nutrition such as *Nutrition For Dummies,* Hungry Minds, Inc., or you can also take a look at Web sites from the American Heart Association (www.american-heart.org) or the American Dietetic Association (www.eatright.org).

I'm not demanding that you try to flip-flop your eating habits starting tomorrow. I just want to nudge you to start thinking twice when you fill your grocery cart or peruse the menu in a restaurant.

Sleeping well

Okay, a show of hands, please: How many of you get enough sleep most of the time? Just as I suspected. Feeling a little sleep-deprived? Doesn't everybody at least some of the time?

If so, you may have a hard time finding the time and energy for your T'ai Chi practice. Your sleepiness makes you want to just flop in a chair like a big sack of beans even if the T'ai Chi moves are gentle. Or a little meditation may find you drifting off rather than drifting inward.

Even with all the alleged time-saving devices, such as e-mail and cell phones, people are running faster and faster, jamming more and more into each day, and trying to squeeze 26 or 28 hours into a mere 24, which in turn infringes on your sleep — if you let it.

You probably know how much sleep you need to feel good. Count back the number of hours of sleep you need from the time you have to get up. Then try to get to bed at the right time so that you can actually enjoy the day, function at 100 percent at work, and still feel good about finding time for some T'ai Chi.

Standing up straight (Your mom was right)

Whether you're meditating or standing in line at the bank, if you stand up tall, you not only feel more confident, but you can also "unkink" your energy channels and let your chi flow more freely. (I discuss these energy channels, called meridians, and the concept of chi more thoroughly in Chapters 13 and 14. Find more details about chi in Chapter 3, too.) Your mama probably didn't know how right she was when she nagged you about standing up straight.

Standing tall doesn't mean maintaining a strained military posture, just keeping a relaxed and spine-straight position. Take a look at the description and figure in Chapter 8 for a good T'ai Chi Posture. Standing straight makes you think more clearly, focus more easily, and meditate better.

Sticking to a sane work schedule

This crazy world sometimes seems to encourage and bless those people who work insane hours, forgoing family, fun, and freedom. Just say no. Doing so doesn't mean becoming a slouch, it just means that you know when enough is enough and when to go home or to take a day off. Work isn't a substitute for other entertainment — you need to go have some non-work-related fun whether you're the CEO or the gofer. Work is only one part of your life. Balance keeps people sane. (For more on this subject, see the principle on balance in Chapter 7.)

Staying healthy and fit

T'ai Chi does a lot for your overall fitness and health. But you may also need — depending on your fitness level or health — to add a few other things to make it a well-rounded program. More stretching, strength-training, or even aerobic exercise, such as brisk walks, can help you achieve more balanced health.

Chapter 17

Trying Mini-Forms

. . . .

In This Chapter

▶ Picking and choosing your goals

▶ Sticking to balance

▶ Working on strength

▶ Flexing your flexibility

▶ Stilling your mind

▶ Conditioning your heart and lungs

. . . .

Sometimes, a full T'ai Chi practice can take your day over the top. Stressfully scrambling to squeeze in your T'ai Chi routine may do the opposite of centering and releasing the flow of your chi. Even the shortest of short forms can be too long — in total minutes or in the concentration demanded, especially if you are learning the movements.

The funny thing is, what is commonly called the Yang Short Form presented in Chapters 9 through 11 is said to have been created partly to fit into busy lifestyles and, at the same time, maintain the beauty and benefits of T'ai Chi. In the decades since the short form was introduced, modern society has jam-packed its days even more. Maybe we need a Yang Short Form Lite?

Instead of Yang Lite (an eight-movement, shortest of short forms is now pro-moted in China), I show you five mini-combinations that are mostly a couple simple forms from the Yang Short Form. They are isolated and combined so you can get your daily T'ai Chi dose without overdosing on stress. Each mini-form — conjured up with the help of my collaborator and instructor Manny — targets a particular goal.

No matter how short your time or how compact the forms you choose to do, always remember the basic principles that I present in Chapter 7. These con-cepts of stillness, slowness, balance, and so on are especially important to focus on when you have only a few minutes to achieve your chi flow. Just slamming out the moves doesn't do you any good, unless all you're interested in is checking T'ai Chi off your to-do list. But that is just so un-T'ai Chi like.

Choosing Goals for Your Mini-Forms

I target five areas with these mini-forms, which apply to everyday activities as well as to sports and fitness endeavors. These areas — which aren't the only ones possible, mind you — are the following:

- **Balance:** Staying upright and walking steadily, not wobbling or and risking spraining an ankle

- **Strength:** Having powerful muscles and connective tissue that can handle tough challenges

- **Flexibility:** Having pliable muscles and soft tissues that bend and flex to keep you injury-free

- **Stillness:** Being quiet and calm and just being with yourself

- **Aerobic conditioning:** Having a strong heart and lungs that can move blood and oxygen faster and more efficiently

In the five mini-forms in this chapter, you use mostly forms, warm-ups, and other movements that I present in other chapters. I refer you to the detailed instructions in such cases, but including here only what you need to be able to understand the concept behind each mini-form. If the movement isn't included in another chapter, I provide you with complete instructions.

Trying the Mini-Tai Chi Forms

These combos are only the beginning! You can put together two or three forms, warm-ups, or movements to fit your needs, schedule, abilities, or preferences. The only thing that limits you — after you get the ideas — is your imagination, which I hope doesn't limit you at all.

Mini-form #1 — Begging for balance

T'ai Chi itself is one big balance drill. Just moving into, through, and out of a Bow Stance (find that basic of all basics in Chapter 8) is a true test of your anti-wobbling ability.

So here I give you one suggestion for working even more specifically on balance: Walk the T'ai Chi Walk. In other words, simply walk T'ai Chi style — which means being slow, flowing, focused, and stabilized, while still applying all the principles that I describe in Chapter 7.

Along with the balance that comes from slow, deliberate T'ai Chi Walking, you also develop leg strength. You stop relying on momentum to get around, and instead appreciate each step. Oh, and one more thing: You practice the basic Centering Step (see Chapter 8) in this mini-form, because that's where the balance part comes in.

You may want to pick a long hallway, large room, or a driveway so that you have plenty of room in front of you to move before you have to break the flow and turn around.

1. **Stand with your heels together, feet turned out slightly to create an angle of about 45 degrees between your toes. Your arms stay relaxed at your sides. If that feels funny, you can place your hands on your hips or waist.**

   If you do this step with your hands on your waist, work toward relaxing them at your sides. Having your arms hang relaxed at your sides makes the walk unstable and, therefore, more challenging because you have to keep your arms from flapping around.

2. **Inhale and then exhale as you bend your right knee, allowing your weight to sink lower on your right leg. Make sure that you feel grounded and stable.**

   Tuck your tailbone under as you sink lower so you don't end up swaying your back and sticking your butt out. That means you should relax your tailbone downward while avoiding collapsing over your ribs and pelvis. (Your posture should still look normal.)

   Now comes the walking stuff.

3. **Inhale and slowly lift your left foot; then, just as slowly, put your left foot down in front of you and slightly to the left of your body as you exhale. Let the heel touch the floor first, and slowly roll down onto the entire sole of the foot. Allow your weight to shift onto the left side while you bend your left knee.**

   This should feel and look nearly like a regular walking step but in slow motion. Also, make sure that your forward-stepping foot doesn't slam down to the ground, but rolls down from the ball of the foot to the heel smoothly and quietly.

4. **When you are finished wobbling on the left leg and feeling nice and stable, inhale and pick up the right foot; then exhale and place the toes lightly on the ground beside your left ankle. (This is the Centering Step discussed in Chapter 8.) Do not move your right foot into the Centering Step position until you are completely wobble-free and well-rooted on the full sole of the front (left) foot.**

You wobble less if you not only sink well, but use your abdominal muscles for centering strength.

5. **Now step out to the right side of your body — just slightly — with your right foot, making sure that the heel goes down first and you roll smoothly and quietly onto the entire foot (no ker-thunks onto the ground!). Use the same transition through the Centering Step, as described in Step 4.**

6. **Continue walking the T'ai Chi Walk until you run out of room; then turn around and head back the way you came. You move in a zigzag fashion, stepping slightly out to one side of your body and then out to the other.**

Avoid lunging forward onto your front leg with a bent knee. Practice putting the heel out in front of you without moving the rest of your body then bringing it back underneath you. You should not have to push off with your front leg to return the foot to the starting position. Only step as far as you can without lunging forward with your weight. Doing the T'ai Chi Walk isn't about Jolly Green Giant steps!

Got all that walking down pat? Now that you can move forward, try doing the walk backward. For example, you can walk forward the length of a hallway and then stop, throw it in reverse, and do the walk going backward, making sure, of course, that there are no tippy lamps or little children behind you.

Mini-forms #2, #3, and #4 — Seeking strength

Let's be frank: I'm not talking about built-up bodies the likes of Arnold here. I'm talking about functional strength — lean and toned muscles that do what you want, when you want, and have enough tone and conditioning to not get hurt or leave you stranded in a pinch.

Know too that the strength required or fostered in T'ai Chi is not brute muscular force, but is the type that comes from within. When you practice unified movements with a relaxed body and a still mind, you find a strength that you perhaps didn't know existed.

Honing leg strength (Horse Stance and Bow Stance)

All of T'ai Chi nurtures strength and endurance in your legs and hips, especially when you sink lower into your knees, which places more challenging demands on your lower body. Although every form works on leg strength, perhaps the best single focus on legs is in basic stance training. Practicing the following stances quickly reminds you that T'ai Chi is not for wimps:

> ✔ **Riding the Horse Stance (mini-form #2):** Your feet are parallel and shoulder-width apart. (See Chapter 8.)
>
> ✔ **Bow Stance (mini-form #3):** This is the basic bow-and-arrow position that in some ways resembles a lunge. (See Chapter 8.)

You can perform these stances with various arm positions just for fun, but if your focus is leg strength, don't let your tiring arms take away from the powerful work happening in your legs. You may — especially at first — want to leave your arms at your sides or let your hands simply rest on your hips.

In the early stages of his T'ai Chi training, Manny recalls arriving at class about 30 minutes early. Alone in the park, he practiced only his stances. He says, "It paid big dividends in strength and stamina. I could make it through classes that usually ran three or four hours."

Attacking arm strength (Standing Like A Tree — #4)

Pushing your body weight around, such as when you do pushups or hoist an iron bar over your head, is one thing. But being able to keep your arms lifted in the air, whether they're moving or not, is truly another matter.

That's what T'ai Chi calls for, so while doing the forms, you target your arms. But to get a foot up (arm up?) you can throw in some standing Qigong-style meditations (such as Standing Like a Tree) that force you to keep your arms lifted and steady. (See Chapters 13 and 14 for more information on Qigong.)

Practicing these meditations gives you one big twofer. You are not only strengthening your arms so that you can better perform the Yang Short Forms (see Chapters 9 through 11), but you're also learning to meditate for an everlasting period. That, in turn, hones your inner power and inner peace.

For the details on arm positions, turn to Chapter 14. Here, I focus strictly on the Embrace the Tree arm position.

1. **Pick a comfortable standing position, perhaps a simple T'ai Chi Posture (see Chapter 8).**

2. **Place your arms in the Embrace the Tree position. Hold for five breath cycles — five inhalations and five exhalations. Lower the arms to rest for a few seconds.**

3. **Alternate holding the position for five breath cycles and then lowering your arms for a brief rest. Do this for up to 10 minutes, or as long as you can.**

Each week (or two, depending on how often you practice), add five breath cycles to your holding position before you lower to rest. In alternating weeks, keep the extended hold, but add five minutes. In other words, you increase the length of your hold one week; then you increase the time that you practice the hold-rest pattern.

Continue to stack these increases until you reach up to an hour of holding without the need to lower to rest.

You may not feel the need to work up to an hour of holding. That's okay. Work up to 10, 20, or 30 minutes instead. The payoff in benefits is proportional to the effort expended, but you can certainly develop sufficient strength and stamina to do good T'ai Chi from being able to hold the arm position for 10 or 15 minutes.

Mini-forms #5, #6, and #7 — Finding flexibility

In a soft and nontargeted way, T'ai Chi can also improve flexibility, especially in your trunk, hips, back, and legs. No, you won't be doing the splits anytime soon, but do you really need to?

For better flexibility, you can add the following three mini-forms to your repertoire, repeating them as needed or as time and space allow.

Lunging-Side-to-Side (#5)

This is the warm-up movement described in Chapter 8. By taking a wide stance and sort of sliding your hips back and forth, you stretch not only your hips but also your inner thighs and legs.

Kick with Left Heel — Kick with Right Heel (#6)

These movements are explained in Chapter 10, where you can also find Figures 10-4 and 10-6 to help you along. For the best stretch, do the movements slowly, lifting each leg as high as you can while keeping good body position. If you want, you can do this mini-form without the arms and hands so that you can focus on the leg and lower body position. These kicks fine-tune balance and leg strength.

1. **Start in a good T'ai Chi Posture (see Chapter 8).**

2. **Step into the first Kick with Heel, choosing one side to start.**

   Be sure to inhale before you start and be sure to exhale with the kicks.

3. **After your foot has reached its peak, lower it slowly to the floor and put your weight on it, shifting your body so your opposite foot lifts off the ground and you're in a Centering Step (see Chapter 8).**

4. **From the Centering Step, do the Kick with Heel on the opposite side.**

5. **Repeat this sequence.**

   You move slightly forward with each kick.

A little bonus to this sequence is the balance *and* leg strength that the kicks help fine-tune.

Snake Creeps Down into Rooster Stands on One Leg — Left and Right (#7)

Here's one movement that you can do slightly out of sequence to repeat it on each side repetitively. Follow these steps and repeat it on both sides several times as one moving sequence.

1. **Begin in the concluding Single Whip position (see Chapter 10 and Figure 10-1) with the right hand in the Dropped Hand position (see Chapter 8) and the left hand pushing out to the side.**

2. **Perform Snake Creeps Down Left into Rooster Stands on Left Leg (see Chapter 11 and Figure 11-1.) Your left hand passes back across the body and down past the right thigh. You end in the one-legged Rooster stance on your left leg.**

3. **Step your right, or lifted, foot forward and move into a transition of the same Single Whip that you started with, but on the opposite side: Your *left* hand is in the Dropped Hand position and your *right* hand is pushing out to the side.**

   Because your primary focus here is on flexibility, don't worry about the exactness of the hand positions at first.

4. **Creep and stand on the other side: Do Snake Creeps Down Right into Rooster Stands on Right Leg (see Chapter 11 and Figure 11-2). Your right hand passes back across your body and down past your left thigh. You end in the one-legged Rooster stance, but this time on your right leg.**

5. **Repeat this sequence, moving from a Single Whip transition into the Creeping Snake on one side and into a Single Whip transition. Then do the Creeping Snake on the other side — until you run out of room. You can then turn around and repeat the mini-form in the opposite direction, if you want.**

Mini-form #8 — Seeking stillness (Standing Like a Tree)

For quieting the mind, calming the body, and developing chi, nothing surpasses standing meditation practice. (For this mini-form, refer to Standing Like a Tree in Chapter 8.) It can give you an even better (and more peaceful) kick-start to your day than that cuppa joe. You can also use standing meditation to give yourself a little stress-free oasis in your day. (Try the bathroom stall at your office if you have to — who will be the wiser?) And this mini-form is a fine way to unwind at day's end.

Any time is a meditative time, but dawn and dusk are the tops:

- **Dawn:** Yang energy of the day begins to grow, and yin energy of the night begins to wane at dawn. (For more information on yin and yang, see the "Opposites Attract: Yin and Yang" sidebar in Chapter 3.) Practicing in the morning allows you to greet the day with a fresh, open, and relaxed mind, ready to face whatever the day brings.
- **Dusk:** Yang energy dissipates, while yin energy grows as the sun sets. Practicing in the evening allows the accumulated mental sludge and sediment to settle or even drift away so that you can enjoy a peaceful evening.

You can find the Standing Like a Tree meditation, which has several variations, in Chapter 14. Do your daily meditation with several arm positions, or alternate one each day.

If you tend to like one arm positions the least, why not start your week with that one?

Aiming for Aerobic Conditioning

T'ai Chi is usually practiced slowly so that you can fully embrace and appreciate the principles. But that's not to say that it can't be done more quickly — or that it hasn't been done at a faster pace, because at its roots, T'ai Chi is a form of combat training. (See Chapters 5 and 6 for more details on T'ai Chi history.) If you were in battle, you'd be moving to save your life — literally.

You can do any of the forms, alone or in combinations of two or three. But a few guidelines apply before you can start doing T'ai Chi in the faster-paced style of Alvin and the Chipmunks.

- **Know the form or forms you intend to do so that you can flow through them without stopping.** That means being able to do them slowly and pretty well before you move it up a notch.
- **Warm up well.** Usually, T'ai Chi is slow enough that you may not need a true warm-up. But you need a warm-up if you're speeding things up. Do the warm-up movements described in Chapter 8. Also, you can do the forms slowly first as a second part of your warm-up.
- **Keep your movements precise.** Don't get sloppy just because you are moving faster. If you can't keep the precision, slow down a tad to a speed where you can still do the movements correctly.

✔ **Start your up-tempo practice moderately.** In other words, don't go as fast as you can at the outset. When you first start trying some speed, go just a little faster than you normally do. Then you can increase the speed one small gear at a time.

✔ **Do a cool-down.** If you move faster, you also need to repeat the selected forms slowly as a way to cool-down. Then you can do some of the warm-up movements as a cool-down, too.

Some Yang Short Forms can work well at a faster pace. You can do them all in place or traveling across the room:

✔ Grasp the Bird's Tail (see Chapter 9)

✔ Wave Hands Like Clouds (see Chapter 10)

✔ Brush Knees (see Chapter 9)

✔ Kick with Left Heel and Kick with Right Heel (see Chapter 10)

✔ Parting the Horse's Mane (see Chapter 9)

Chapter 18

Taking a Moment for Qigong

In This Chapter

▶ Refreshing yourself with Qigong mini-breaks

▶ Tapping into your energy

▶ Stimulating your organs

▶ Finding peace while standing

*P*racticing Qigong doesn't have to take a long time. If you want to take breaks during your day, you can do some stances and chi-stimulating movements in a few minutes. Take a look at Chapter 14 for some introductory Qigong movements you can try whenever a mini-moment strikes.

But even though some Qigong moves take only a few minutes, they may leave you a bit baffled. Which one should I do? When? Why? I suggest that you lay out a few moves with specific goals so you can grab them and practice as needed.

In this chapter, I give you five Qigong mini-breaks. I often refer you to Chapter 14. If necessary, I refer you to the instructions in the other chapters, but I include the crux of the forms here so you can work your way through them without getting confused. If the movement is new, I give you instructions. The new moves are simple, so don't be alarmed.

Qigong is another internal martial art that emphasizes tapping into your energy and releasing its flow in your body. Get the energy moving, it is said, and you'll be healthier, happier, and develop a better T'ai Chi practice to boot. (I introduce Qigong in Chapter 6, and I explain it in more detail in Chapter 13, with more information on movements and meditations in Chapter 14.)

Note that I use a couple movements from The Eight Treasures (see Chapter 14). Traditionally, you practice these eight movements in one session and in the particular order described in Chapter 14 to reap the most benefits. But even though I isolate a couple of The Eight Treasures for Qigong mini-breaks, benefits still abound. I promise that the wrath of the heavens won't come down on you for not doing them all together.

Scoring with Quick Qigong Goals

Certainly, you can do these mini-breaks as a part of a longer routine or for other reasons, but you can do them for three common reasons:

✔ **To refresh yourself:** Who doesn't sometimes need a pick-me-up? That may be first thing in the morning, during a coffee break, or after work — make it a Qigong break! A little boost of energy recirculation can refresh and rejuvenate you.

✔ **To relieve stress:** If you need refreshment, you sometimes need to rid a little stress, too. With the right movement, you can help yourself feel less anxious and more peaceful.

✔ **To eliminate bad chi:** You want a flow of chi, but it needs to be good chi. You can pick up bad chi from other people, stress, or poor health. Getting rid of bad chi leaves room for the good stuff to fill you up.

Trying the Qigong Mini-Breaks

These movements are only the beginning! You can put together two or three movements and do them for as long or as short as you need to. And the more practice you get, the better you become at finding the refreshing and relieving rewards after practicing a short time. If you have a little creativity, you can Qigong and Qigong some more. (In Chapter 19, you can find a few examples of combining Tai Chi and Qigong even for more variety in your mini-breaks.)

Let the Qigong-ing begin! (I know that's not a word, but doesn't it have a nice ring?)

Mini-breaks #1 and #2 — Refreshing and energizing

Nearly all the Qigong movements refresh you in some way. Here are a couple suggestions geared toward that specific goal.

Slapping, Rubbing, and Looking Behind You (#1)

If you take any Qigong, you may be asked to hit yourself. Wait, what? At my first Qigong class, I was a bit taken aback by the slapping and rubbing, but I followed suit. When in Rome, do as the Romans do, huh? I was surprised to realize how good it felt. You will too.

Like a massage, the rubbing and slapping stimulates circulation and flushes out the muscles. These movements can also stimulate the flow of chi.

1. **Stand in good Qigong Posture (also known as good Tai Chi Posture, as described in Chapter 8).**

2. **Perform Looking Behind You (#4) from The Eight Treasures routine. Take a look at Chapter 14.**

3. **Return to a simple Qigong Posture, and use your hands to gently slap yourself all over your body, trying to cover as much as you can with your palms. Include your neck, shoulders, arms, buttocks, and legs — every part that you can get to.**

   If you want, try gentle and quick rubbing after you've gently slapped yourself, or sort of alternate between rubbing and slapping.

4. **Settle back into a good Qigong Posture, and repeat the Looking Behind You move, followed by the slapping and rubbing.**

   Repeat these two movements as many times as you want.

Three-part Energizer (#2)

This mini-break isn't in Chapter 14, so I give you careful details here. Manny, my collaborator, often does this movement during his regular T'ai Chi classes. (See Chapters 6 and 13 for information about the relationship between T'ai Chi and Qigong.) This mini-break has three parts, so be sure to do them all and in order for the best energizing reward.

You can do this energizer at several different times:

- ✔ At the end of your warm-up but before you start your forms or stances.

- ✔ At the end of your class or practice to reenergize.

- ✔ At any time, especially when you realize that you've been sitting too long. (Hmm, I wonder if it can be done in airplane bathrooms? Nah.)

Taking time to breathe

1. **Start in good Tai Chi Posture (see Chapter 8). Remember that your knees are bent, but bend them only as much as is comfortable. Hold your hands in front of you, resting slightly against your thighs, as if you are holding a really heavy stack of books. Your arms are nearly straight, and your fingers are pointed in toward each other, almost touching.**

2. **Inhale and let your arms swing out to your sides and upward, almost as if you are doing a super slow jumping jack without moving your feet. When your arms reach shoulder-height, rotate your palms so they face upward; the arms continue to rise until they are just above**

your head (like the "Y" in movements to the song "YMCA"). Feel your body lift and float upward as your arms rise, but don't let your knees straighten completely. Stay grounded so you can suck up all the chi you can.

Try to coordinate your breathing and arm-raising so you run out of breath about the same time that your arms reach the top.

3. **Pause for a second at the top. Slowly rotate your palms to face out-ward. Then exhale slowly and fully as you sink your body back into your knees and return your hands to the starting position on your thighs in front of you.**

4. **Repeat this 4–6 times, or as many as 10–12 times before moving on to the second part.**

Stimulating the internal organs

I love Manny's analogy for the second part of this energizer: This part is like shaking a bottle of soda, except your body is the bottle, so you're going to shake, baby, shake, gyrate, and jiggle.

Here's the scoop on this shaking stuff. In the West, people are always concerned about the external muscles — how they look, how they feel, if they're lean or sized right, and so on. In fact, when you do traditional Western-style aerobic exercise (think jogging or cycling), your blood flow actually passes by your inner organs and heads off to the working muscles. That's just the opposite of what happens in the Eastern arts because the internal organs and their proper working is key.

This second part focuses on your innards. You may see similarities between this movement and parts of The Eight Treasures movements detailed in Chapter 14.

1. **Stand in the traditional Tai Chi Posture (see Chapter 8). Let your arms hang loosely, naturally, and comfortably at your sides.**

Keep your entire upper body loose and relaxed throughout this exercise. Your arms flop freely, and your facial muscles may even jiggle if you're relaxed enough! Don't worry — no one is watching.

2. **Rise up on your toes and then drop your heels to the floor quickly. Do this exercise rapidly. Don't think about carefully lowering your heels, as if you were afraid of crushing some eggs. Instead, think about rapidly dropping your heels to the floor, as if you want to crush an egg or two. Repeat these drops for 10–15 seconds.**

Your knees remain in the same slightly bent position the whole time you rise and drop. The entire movement is in the feet and ankles. Everything above your feet and ankles is just going along for the rather bumpy ride.

Don't be concerned with extremes. Don't try to go up as high as you possibly can, but go up just high enough to get a good drop. That may be only about half of your possible rise. Your heels strike the ground firmly at the end of each drop.

3. **Rise up one last time on your toes a little higher and slower, and drop your heels down to the ground very sharply.**

   This is one set. Done properly, you start to feel a tingling sensation in your palms of your hands at the end of each set because of the increased energy flow being moved up your legs and through your body.

4. **Do 4–5 sets, or as many as 10–12, if you have time. Remember that you are shaking it all up, so let it go.**

If you have problems with your back, wear special orthotics, or have any foot problems such as plantar fasciitis or heel spurs, don't do this part unless your physician approves it.

Massaging your insides, too

When you get a massage, it feels good, doesn't it? Just imagine how good it feels to massage your internal organs! You not only get the same good feelings as with an outer-body massage, but you also stimulate blood flow and free the flow of chi.

1. **Stand with your feet parallel and the insides of your ankles touching. Bend your knees slightly and lean your body forward about 45 degrees from the hips.**

   To protect your back, keep your spine straight. Don't slump over from the lower back, but bend from your hip joints, as if you are folding in half.

   Here comes the massage part.

2. **In the leaned-over position, imagine that a rope is slung across your shoulders and hanging down on both sides. Pretend use the ends of the rope to lift buckets out of a well. But don't use your arms — let them just hang there like limp spaghetti noodles. Pretend that they don't exist. Raise one shoulder and then the other, alternating one going up while the other goes down. Your body wiggles like a silly snake.**

3. **Continue this movement — slowly — for a couple minutes.**

   Assuming that you don't lean over too far, this movement can be good for your back. But if you have back problems, make sure that you get a physician's clearance. Manny suffered a back problem many years ago, and says that this movement has helped keep his back loose, stretched, and strengthened.

Mini-breaks #3 and #4 — Relieving stress

Do I really need to explain the glories of relieving stress? Nope, I didn't think so. So I cut straight to the quick and move into the explanations for two more Qigong mini-breaks

Standing and Finding Peace (#3)

One of the great benefits of a Qigong practice is how well it can help make stress drift away. Stress in the body often comes from muscle tension. A little Qigong can relax tense muscles and, therefore, lead to long-lasting and deep muscle and mental relaxation.

This mini-break simply refers to another movement in this book. But as the simplest and shortest of the mini-breaks, it shows you how crucial standing peacefully can be.

To do Standing and Finding Peace, take a look at Standing Like a Tree, as well as a few possible hand positions, in Chapter 14.

You don't have to do this mini-break in tandem with any routine. Whether you have 5 minutes or 30 minutes, you can stand like a tree. Have you ever seen a stressed-out tree?

Meditation practice allows you to focus on one point and allows distracting, stressful thoughts to fall away. By practicing this exercise on a daily basis, you can develop a sort-of bubble of serenity that envelops you and goes with you — wherever you go.

So be the tree and find your bubble of serenity.

Jolting and Wagging (#4)

For this mini-break, you do two of The Eight Treasures (see Chapter 14). Heck, you can even do just one of them. Personally, I have a soft spot for Wagging My Head and Tail.

1. **Do 3–6 repetitions of Bending Over and Wagging Head and Tail (#5) from The Eight Treasures routine. You can do more if you want.**

2. **Do several repetitions of Jolting the Back of the Body (#8) from The Eight Treasures routine.**

Be sure to do a balanced number of each movement. In other words, don't do nine Wagging but only one Jolting.

Mini-break #5 — Getting rid of bad chi

Much of Qigong practice is mental, relying on imagery and tapping into your mind. You can successfully free your chi, dump the bad stuff, and find peace if you believe that these things can happen. This believing bit can be hard for the left-brained, just-the-facts kind of person. But maybe that's who should be doing all these movements.

If you feel that your chi is somewhat stagnant — like a creek going dry in the summer — this quick movement can help you with the flow.

1. **Start in good Tai Chi Posture (see Chapter 8). Knees remain slightly bent during this movement. Let your arms and hands hang relaxed at your sides.**

2. **Inhale and raise your hands in front of you to shoulder-height during the inhalation. Keep your hands shoulder-width apart. Your palms face up. The elbows stay a little bent and point toward the floor.**

3. **When your hands reach shoulder-height, pull them in to your shoulders (right to right and left to left) while turning your palms gently away from you so they face forward.**

This movement is smooth and steady. It flows from your hands hanging down to lifting up to pulling in. If it were a sentence, it wouldn't have any punctuation.

4. **Exhale and push your hands forward and away from your body during the exhalation. Then return your hands to their starting position by your sides.**

Here's where the mind kicks in: When you lift your hands and inhale, imagine yourself gathering good and fresh chi up and into you, with your hands and with your breath. When you rotate your palms out and exhale as you push away, imagine yourself pulling bad chi from your body and shoving it out of your life. Also see yourself expelling the stagnant chi with your breath.

5. **Do this movement for a few minutes, or for as long as you feel is necessary.**

Chapter 19

Combining Qigong and T'ai Chi

T'ai Chi and Qigong have a lot to offer the willing and diligent practitioner. Although these practices are usually practiced as separate disciplines, they can be combined in different ways to develop high levels of chi and good health. In this chapter, I give you some suggestions on how you can combine T'ai Chi and Qigong into your practice. As you get deeper into your practice, you may find combinations of your own that address your needs. Don't be afraid to experiment as you gain the knowledge to feel comfortable doing so.

Deciding What You Want to Gain

Depending on your intent, you can put together mini-combos of T'ai Chi and Qigong based on two concepts:

- ✔ **Similarity:** You want to develop stillness, or balance, or grounding or some particular concept, so you choose movements from T'ai Chi and Qigong that work on that one principle for extra reinforcement and practice.

- ✔ **Contrast:** You want to work on your ability to flow between types of movements, such as yin (softer) and yang (more energetic) movements (see Chapter 3). So you put together a couple moves that allow you to work on the contrast of the types and your ability to move from one feeling to another.

Doing It Your Mini-Combo Way

You know the advertising tunes about doing it your way. The same thing applies to the T'ai Chi–Qigong combos put together here for you to sample. These examples are a good place to start. But after you get the idea, I encourage you to do it your way! Put together two, three, or four movements or warm-ups to fit your needs, schedule, or ability. Choose ones that you like, and choose ones that seem a little difficult for you. Or choose ones that are similar or contrasting.

I provide instructions and figures in Chapters 8 through 11, and 14 for the forms that are also in this chapter. When these forms come up, I describe any necessary transitions and then refer you to the appropriate chapter and figure so you can flip back easily. For the new forms, I present all the instruction here. You also find references to the basic concepts in other chapters to help you fully grasp the meaning and teachings.

Mini-combo #1 — Yearning for yin and yang

This combination incorporates two things:

The opposing "yin" and "yang" in the advancing (yang) and retreating (yin) movements in Grasp the Bird's Tail of the Yang Short Form presented in Chapters 9-11.

The yin and yang of the Grasp Tail movement partnered with the stillness (yin) of a Qigong-oriented meditative stance focused on gathering your chi. (Take a look at Chapter 3 and 13 for more on that.)

Grasp the Bird's Tail and Riding the Horse chi meditation

Alternate Grasp the Bird's Tail on one side with a Riding the Horse stance focused on your Dan Tien. (See Chapter 13 for more information on the Dan Tien.)

1. **Grasp the Bird's Tail — Right five times. You can find the instruction and figures illustrating this form in Chapter 9.**

   One way to do this move repetitively is to move your rear foot from the concluding Push position next to your front foot into a Centering Step. You can then simply switch feet in the Centering Step and then progress into your next Grasp the Bird's Tail on the same side.

Try to do this little ditty without the basic Centering Step between the repetitions. Why? If you stay rooted in the Bow Stance and remove the little rest break, you make your legs stronger and avoid interrupting the flow of chi.

Although I suggest doing this movement five times, you can do more or less, depending on your time or ability.

2. **Sit back with your body weight on your left leg, being sure to bend the knee and sink. Pivot your right foot inward on the heel, turning your body to the left so you end up in a Riding the Horse stance, as I discuss in Chapter 8. Adjust your left foot so it is also turned straight ahead and is parallel to the right foot.**

Make sure that you don't have any weight on the leg of the foot that is pivoting so you don't hurt your knees or hips. And only pivot as far as you are comfortable.

3. **As you move into the stance, bring your hands in front of your chest in an Embrace the Tree position, which is explained in Chapter 14.**

4. **Imagine that the "tree" is shrinking into a smaller ball about the size of a volleyball. Your arms and elbows float to your sides so you can hold this ball between your hands in front of your Dan Tien, or about at your navel, with your fingers pointing away from you. Hold this position.**

After you understand the Dan Tien position, you can go straight to it as you pivot into the Riding the Horse stance without starting in the Embrace the Tree position.

5. **Inhale slowly and fully. Imagine the chi gathering in your Dan Tien. As you exhale slowly and fully, imagine the chi travelling into the imaginary ball that you are holding, filling it full of energy. Breathe in and out five times.**

6. **Repeat the process, this time doing Grasp the Bird's Tail — Left. Shift your weight onto the left leg and then pivot your right foot inward on the heel. Shift your weight back onto your right leg and then step out with your left foot into a Bow Stance. Follow the instructions for Grasp the Bird's Tail — Left in Chapter 9.**

7. **Do up to five repetitions of Grasp the Bird's Tail — Left and follow the pivot transition explained in Step 2 to get into the Qigong stance. Then repeat Steps 3 through 5.**

You can continue to alternate the Grasp Tail form with the Riding the Horse stance as long as you want.

Avoid hurrying the repetitions. If staying longer or doing more feels good, by all means, do so!

Mini-combo #2 — Orbiting cosmically

This combination combines the powerful lateral movement of Wave Hands Like Clouds with a Qigong movement that helps you move your chi through the body and its microcosmic orbit. (You can find an explanation of the microcosmic orbit in Chapter 13.)

Wave Hands Like Clouds and Microcosmic Orbit

Like the first mini-combo, you alternate movements. This time, however, you move between the lateral dynamics of Wave Hands Like Clouds and the stationary but potent microcosmic orbit meditation.

1. **Wave Hands Like Clouds, first moving to your left for five steps. (Refer to Chapter 10.)**

2. **Step your left foot out and into a good posture, which for Qigoing is the same as the T'ai Chi Posture (refer to Chapter 8).**

   The stance for a good posture is not wide but one where your feet are about shoulder-width apart with your weight centered over them.

3. **Move into a microcosmic orbit meditation (see Chapter 14).** For more details on what the microcosmic orbit is, take a look at Chapter 13.)

4. **Return to Wave Hands Like Clouds, this time moving to your right for five steps. Follow this step with a standing microcosmic orbit meditation.**

   You can continue these movements — laterally waving along and then punctuating the movement with a standing meditation — as long as you want or need.

Mini-combo #3 — Developing chi

This combination uses the traditional opening of the Yang Short Form for its grounding balance before moving into more chi development through both a T'ai Chi and a Qigong movement. If you want to read more about chi, refer to Chapters 3 and 13.

Commencement, Parting the Horse's Mane, and Qigong Walking

Compared to the first two mini-combos that use two movements, this one uses three so you can have another option to try as you put together your own ideas. Each movement in this mini-combo is different and forces you to focus so that your chi doesn't scatter, especially when you transition between them.

1. **Start with the traditional Commencement, or Opening the Door, movement (see Chapter 9 for details). Use the upward and downward chi-gathering movements to focus yourself as you begin.**

2. **Concentrate on the yin and the yang of the hands rising and body sinking and then the hands sinking and the body rising. Do the movement five times, inhaling as the hands rise and exhaling as they sink.**

   I prescribe a certain number of repetitions, but you can always increase or decrease your movements. This number isn't carved in stone.

3. **When you finish your opening repetitions, shift your weight to your right leg to move into a Centering Step (see Chapter 8 for information on the basic steps). At the same time, your arms float into the Hold Balloon position with your right hand on top and left hand on the bottom. (This basic is also described in Chapter 8.)**

4. **Inhale and then exhale as you step out on your left foot to do Parting the Horse's Mane (see Chapter 9)**

   Don't get yourself all tied up in knots about this transition. You can find it laid out in Chapter 9, and it should be easy because Parting the Horse's Mane actually follows the Commencement in the Yang Short Form.

5. **Shift your weight back to the Centering Step with your weight on your right leg and return your arms to the Hold Balloon position. This allows you to repeat Parting the Horse's Mane as many times as you like.**

6. **After your repetitions, shift your weight back to the right leg again, but this time, you're preparing to step out into a Qigong Walk.**

7. **Start your Qigong Walk with your left foot stepping out. Walk very slow five steps with each foot — more if you want, or as many as you can before crashing into a wall.**

   After you finish the walk, you may need to turn around before you repeat the set.

8. **Finish your walk by stepping both feet into your good T'ai Chi — er — Qigong Posture. Now you're ready to repeat the entire set, starting with the Commencement.**

Part VI
The Part of Tens

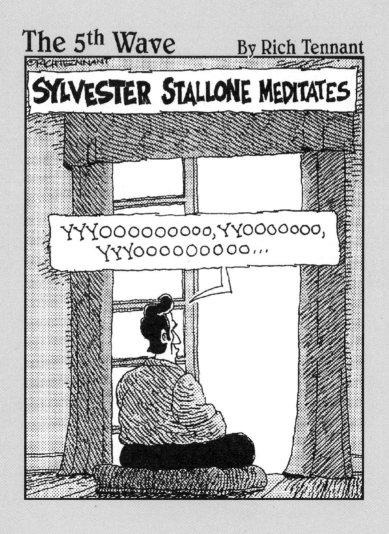

The 5th Wave   By Rich Tennant

SYLVESTER STALLONE MEDITATES

YYYoooooooooo, YYooooooo, YYYooooooooooo...

In this part . . .

This is the fun stuff. The other parts are, too, mind you, but you can flip through and use this stuff at any time, even in daily life. And it's all concise and written in an easy-to-read format. You get bits on T'ai Chi philosophy, some wise quotes, and a segment on Taoist lessons. These lists of tens include some great words that you can peruse time and time again. At first, they may be entertaining. But trust me on this: Go back to these chapters as you advance in your practice, because the advice and suggestions take on different shapes each time you read them. Parts stand out that you didn't notice the first time around — perhaps because you become more familiar with them the second time around, the third time around, and so on.

Chapter 20

Ten Benefits of Practicing T'ai Chi

*P*racticing T'ai Chi — heck, for that matter, Qigong or any of the mindful or internal Chinese movement arts — can help you nail down a whole laundry list of mental and physical benefits.

Some people may not believe that gaining any of these benefits is possible simply by doing some movements that from all outward appearances look pretty simplistic. It's up to you to decide what to believe. Whether you believe in the benefits of T'ai Chi may have some bearing on what you eventually experience in return.

This list of ten benefits isn't all-inclusive. Nor is it all scientifically validated, researched, poked, prodded, and proved. Perhaps many of these benefits may never find the proof they need. (For more detail, including a little foray into what the scientific literature does say — as well as what it doesn't say — take a look at Chapter 2.)

I can't guarantee that you'll experience all these benefits. Nor can I say that you won't experience something else. Everybody is different concerning their weak points and strong points, so what each person gains will be different, too.

Any great stuff that you experience from a T'ai Chi practice has a lot to do with the effort invested. Practice once in a blue moon and maybe only half-heartedly, and you can't get much out of it. Practice diligently and work on proper form, techniques, and all the basics over time, and you may get what's on this list . . . and more.

Reduce Stress and Anxiety

I think that more and more people are getting completely fed up with the faster, more frenzied world in which we live, not to mention frustrated, because slowing down seems so difficult.

T'ai Chi can be an island in the storm. Reducing stress or eliminating anxiety is probably a primary reason many people take to it. Even if you don't get it right away — be that a form's progression or what all the chi stuff means — you'll probably walk away feeling better after even one class. Why? Because slowing down suddenly becomes okay; you can take a breath and find your inner peace.

T'ai Chi is sometimes referred to as "meditation in motion" or "moving meditation." That's not a bad description, either. Even a small amount of meditation can reduce your stress, your anxiety, and your feelings of being overwhelmed.

Clear Your Mind

Mental clarity certainly goes hand-in-hand with reducing stress. Who can be stress-free but still have things banging around inside the head like Ping-Pong balls in a lottery game spin?

With stress reduction comes the ability to clear the mind and bring full attention to the present moment. T'ai Chi is one of many movement practices that unifies mind and body. For other such practices, take a look at *Mind-Body Fitness For Dummies,* by yours truly (Hungry Minds, Inc). This unification brings the body and the mind to the same place at the same time so you can fully experience the present rather than continually live in a swirl of what-if, what-was, what-can-be, or what-may-happen.

If you live in the present moment with a clear mind, you don't wallow in guilt and regret over past events that you can't change. Nor do you live in fear of future events that may — or may not — actually happen.

Improve Your Outlook on Life

Like many activities, T'ai Chi can produce a feeling of accomplishment and success. This alone can help you feel better about yourself and improve how you feel about life. But T'ai Chi goes a step farther than all those other activities. The feelings of accomplishment imparted through a T'ai Chi practice must come from within. They are internally sparked and are about you, instead of being externally produced and brought on perhaps by some performance or comparison to others. Now, I'm not saying that other activities can't produce great feelings because of intrinsic or internal motivators, but T'ai Chi is only about what goes on inside.

The smallest bubble of chi inside can mean that you are successful. Heck, just practicing is a victory on any particular day and leaves you feeling better about all that swirls around you.

Manny says that only two things are required for success in a T'ai Chi practice:

- ✔ Start
- ✔ Continue

What is a simpler way to feel better? Now, you may find it takes you a little longer than just partaking. Everybody is different, of course. But the meditative slow stress-releasing movement can just help you feel better about life's goings-on.

Develop Discipline and Self-Control

Sure, you can join the army, practice piano scales for hours a day, or become addicted to your Day Planner. The point being, T'ai Chi is not the only way to develop more self-discipline.

But T'ai Chi is still a very good way. And, well, I'd choose T'ai Chi over military enlistment or piano scales. What about you?

Practicing regularly helps instill the discipline and dedication to make yourself do things even when you don't feel like it. Unfortunately, we need to do things in life that we don't ever feel much like doing. (Dishwashing anyone?) Part of this is all about habit: Develop a habit, which alone encourages the self-discipline to do the job. The get-up-and-go part that can be hard, but afterward, you're often glad you did.

Okay, this is not to say that you should practice daily, come sickness, injury, pain, or strain. It just means being diligent. The diligence you nurture then carries over into daily life, from being able to stand up for yourself, getting aerobic exercise, not sitting in front of the TV all evening, or turning down second and third helpings when you know that you don't need them.

Achieve Better Health

Now this is something you can sink your teeth into. Better health can mean everything from lower cholesterol and lower blood pressure to diminished lower back pain or less pain and stiffness from arthritis. Sound good?

Your wallet will like this benefit, which can mean fewer bucks going out to pay for doctor bills and more staying in the billfold for fun stuff. The health care system likes this one, too, because it can cut down on the number of sick people who need lots of care. Even your lifestyle will like this one: Better health means that you can get around and enjoy yourself more day-to-day and live a happier, healthier, and higher quality life.

No, T'ai Chi alone may not be enough to completely lower the risk of heart disease and cancers, but the scientific panel is still out on that one. Either way, T'ai Chi certainly doesn't hurt in an attempt to stem the tide of deaths and sickness from lifestyle diseases, such as heart disease, in our technologically advanced society.

But what you really care about is just feeling better — and you will.

Acquire Better Balance

This is another kingpin benefit of regular T'ai Chi practice, and one that is proven by scientific research (see Chapter 2). Whoopee! Science gives the nod of approval.

What I'm talking about is the ability to stay upright. Now, you're thinking that falling is something old people do. Yes, maybe. But unless you train balance, you lose it. And that shows up as fall-down go-boom when you're older. Not old. Just older.

The slow-paced moves, leg raises, and body rotations increase leg strength, body coordination, torso strength, kinesthetic awareness, and *neuromuscular proprioception* (basically, your nerves and muscles communicate better). All put together, you're more confident standing upright. And you can stay upright better.

Breathe Better

In a T'ai Chi practice, you have to think about your breathing. That's something you don't normally do; breathing comes naturally. But breathing fully and deeply may not be. If you breathe fully, with shoulders relaxed and abdomen expanding properly, you get more oxygen in (that's the good stuff) and more carbon dioxide out (that's the bad stuff).

Taking in solid and slow breaths can also lower your heart rate. All together, the heart doesn't have to work as hard to do its job in helping move oxygen along to the rest of the body.

In laymen's terms: A full and deep breath just feels dang good. I suppose that's really all that matters.

Find the Flexibility in Your Muscles

My bet is, you know that your muscles are tighter than they used to be, whether you exercise or not. My bet is, you've leaned over to pick up something off the ground or tied your shoe and said, "Man, I used to be able to do this." Am I right?

Okay then, that may seem like a minor thing to not be able to do, but tight muscles can lead to injury, such as lower back strain, or to pain and discomfort.

The relaxed state and soft but dynamic movements in T'ai Chi promote better flexibility, so you can achieve more range of motion in your joints.

So next time you reach for the floor or your shoe, you'll actually get there.

Perfect Your Posture

If less stress, better balance, or a cheerier outlook on life aren't good enough, how about a tall and strong posture? Compared to some traditional exercises that can promote overly tight muscles that can cause poor posture, T'ai Chi can result in the posture of the century: head erect, shoulders relaxed, chest strong but not puffed out and militaristically tense, back straight, and feet firmly on the floor.

Quite commanding, actually.

Good posture also promotes good energy flow up and down the spine. (There's that chi stuff again. Read more about it in Chapter 3.) What else does good posture do? Keeps your internal organs from being squished up on one another because of slouching or slumping. Promotes a healthier lower back from balanced muscle use. And helps you feel more self-confident!

Lower Your Blood Pressure

Actually, any regular aerobic exercise that raises your heart rate even a small amount can help drop your blood pressure. T'ai Chi isn't alone here. But the addition of mindful breathing and focus of T'ai Chi gives an extra push in that direction.

Of course, this kind of benefit isn't guaranteed, and if you have high blood pressure, you want to talk to your doctor before beginning any exercise program.

Still, wrap up less stress, a lower heart rate, a better outlook on life, more relaxation, better use of oxygen, and a smile on your face, and you may see lower numbers on that blood pressure gauge, too.

Chapter 21

Ten Times and Places to Add a Little T'ai Chi to Your Life

In This Chapter

▶ Scheduling your T'ai Chi moments

▶ Opening your mind to different practice times, like in traffic jams or waiting lines

▶ Using T'ai Chi in beautiful settings, such as mountains or beaches

T'ai Chi isn't just about practicing all the forms in front of your teacher in a classroom. It's also about finding the times that feel best to you and that best suit your needs. Finding that time or place can mean a better flow of chi in your body.

Don't get me wrong. I don't mean that you'll be doing an entire 24-form progression while waiting in a line at the post office. Ooooh, that'd attract a few stares — and could get you to the front of the line sooner, I suppose. But, seriously, this chapter is about seeking little corners in your life where you can fit in just a few minutes, or one or two forms, perhaps because you're stressed and need it or perhaps because it's so beautiful that you're moved to do it.

Take a look at this list for some ideas:

At Sunrise

When the sun starts to bloom over the horizon can be the most idyllic moment not only to practice T'ai Chi but also to think about the power of the earth. Traditional Chinese practitioners hold classes and groups very early so they can take advantage of this time of day. That's because practicing at sunrise can increase your *yang*, or stronger energy, and decrease your *yin*, or softer energy. To get on with your day, getting a dose of yang can be just the right medicine.

At Sunset

Then you've got the sun leaving you as it sinks below the horizon. Sunset is the second most popular — and second most appropriate — time of day to practice. Why? For the opposite reasons as sunrise. At the end of your day, you want to slow down, decrease your yang energy, and increase your yin energy.

Traditionally, practitioners recommend practicing forms at sunrise *and* at sunset. That way, you can fully take advantage of changing your energy not only at the start of your day but also at the end of your day. Not everybody can practice at both times. But I'm not talking about an hour. How about 5 minutes each time on days when you aren't ready to undertake a full practice? It can help you transition into and out of your day better.

When Stress Has a Grip on You

A really good T'ai Chi session requires that your mind is calm and relaxed when you start the session. But with today's modern world, starting your practice blissfully is not always possible. So you can also use your session to get you relaxed when you sense your body starting to seize up from stress or when the cares of the world are starting to pen you in.

I'm not talking about a full-blown practice session. This can be as simple as doing one form — such as Wave Hands Like Clouds — for a few minutes, or maybe just practicing one or more of the standing meditation stances. No matter what you choose to do, a few minutes of T'ai Chi calms your mind and soothes your spirit. (Check out Chapters 9 through 11 for more information on specific T'ai Chi movements.)

While You're on a Long Drive

Now don't get silly. I am not advocating that you close your eyes and do a meditation. The highway patrol probably won't feather to that as an excuse for the accident you've caused. (But officer . . . I was just doing what the book says!)

Driving long distances can take a lot out of you and leave you feeling beat up when you get to your destination. Whenever you take a break to buy a snack or hit the restroom, find a quiet place to practice T'ai Chi for a couple of minutes. No matter which form you choose, or if you even choose some Qigong, you'll likely finish up with a looser back and more relaxed neck and shoulders. And if you're getting the sleepies, a few minutes of chi-stimulating moves (check out Chapters 14 or 18) can help pep you up for another leg of the drive. Likely, you'll arrive feeling more refreshed and energetic.

Sitting in Traffic

Here you go again, imagining that you are jumping out of your car in a traffic jam so you can Grasp the Bird's Tail. Now, really! When you're stuck in your car (or even some boring meeting or class), you can take on a little mental practice, sort of like visualizing your performance.

From athletes and dancers to public speakers and musicians — all use visualization to prepare for the actual event. You can do the same with your T'ai Chi practice. Any time the traffic isn't moving, do some deep abdominal breathing and mentally run through a T'ai Chi form or movement sequence. Picture yourself doing the movements properly, at the right tempo, and using all the principles of T'ai Chi. This is an enormously beneficial practice: Try it sometime when you aren't stuck somewhere, too.

Standing in Line

Anytime you find yourself waiting in line — at the store, at the bank, to buy concert tickets, you name it — you can engage in a little informal T'ai Chi practice. This may not mean putting down your things and doing a few forms. Instead, try finding your good T'ai Chi posture, practice a little full breathing, sink into a meditation stance, feel your acupoints in your feet firmly planted and pulling up energy from the earth, or do little chi-feeling exercises with your hands. (For more on acupoints, turn to Chapter 13.)

Otherwise thought of as wasted time, waiting in line now becomes a few moments to look forward to during a busy day.

In a Park

The absolute best, no-questions-asked, hands-down, winner-take-all place to practice mentally or physically is outdoors. For most people, that means a park. But that can also mean a wonderful backyard. Just think green and trees.

Manny says that a nice park is located across the street from his teacher's house. And that's where they went every Saturday — rain or shine, hot or cold — to practice their forms for about four hours. "There is a special feeling to practicing out in nature, feeling the sun or rain or breeze on your skin, smelling the flowers and fresh air, and enjoying the sounds of birds singing and breezes rustling through the branches of the trees," he says. "And practicing in the same place throughout the year gave me a sense of the cyclical nature of life, as I observed the cycle of birth, growth, death, and decay in the natural world."

Head outdoors. Take time to tune into the energy around you from the thriving trees and green plants. For your standing meditations, seek to emulate the strength and energy of an oak tree — firmly rooted, solid, and strong on the bottom, yet soft and yielding on the top.

At the Beach or Lake

Any waterfront is a great place to practice T'ai Chi because of the power of the sea meeting the land and sky, as well as the energy from lapping or breaking waves and the sense of peace from a rustling breeze. If you're on a sandy waterfront, practicing barefoot can further challenge your ability to move, stay rooted, and keep your balance.

In the Mountains

Like the water, the mountains have power — in most cases, a good energy because you become aware of the primal forces of nature. Whether you have mountains in your backyard, as I do, or you take advantage of the vacation view at the Blue Ridge Mountains, you can ultimately experience the life and energy so key to T'ai Chi. This experience is never truly possible in a classroom.

In Front of a Mirror

No full-length mirrors outdoors, at the beach, or in the mountains, but as you practice T'ai Chi, a little form-checking and posture reality is good for you too.

Walls covered with mirrors provide an excellent way to inspect yourself from all sides. As you know, looking good on the outside is less important than feeling the right thing on the inside. But you may never discover how to feel the right thing unless you practice the right position with the best posture. Sort of a chicken-and-egg thing. Even if you swear by parks, get in front of a mirror now and then. But don't let it become a daily crutch.

Chapter 22

Ten (Plus One) Ways to Supplement Your T'ai Chi Practice

• •

In This Chapter

▶ Letting a little Tao into your life

▶ Taking on videos and books to expand your vision

▶ Practicing mentally and mentally practicing

▶ Applying the principles day in and day out

• •

*P*racticing T'ai Chi is a bit like learning to drive a car. If you learn to drive a small car with an automatic transmission on city streets, you aren't done. You need to add to your driving knowledge so you can become a more well-rounded, smarter, and safer driver. You may also want to drive a truck, a manual transmission, or even a four-wheel drive automobile. You need to drive on some winding roads and perhaps in bad weather. Knowing a little bit about these other things can make you a better driver.

Likewise, in T'ai Chi, you know the short form and maybe a teeny bit of Qigong. Trying or reading about other things can supplement your practice so your T'ai Chi actually becomes better. Take a look at these things, any one of which can help you become a more well-rounded and better T'ai Chi practitioner.

Read a Little Taoism

Taoism (*dow*-ism) is the philosophy underlying T'ai Chi, as well as other Chinese internal martial arts or spiritual and health practices, such as Qigong. Taoism, as a philosophy of going about your life, is not a religion (although it can be a religion practiced in other ways), and it doesn't request that you give up your current beliefs. This kind of Taoism is a way of living in — and looking at — the world harmoniously. It advocates simplicity and selflessness.

With that kind of emphasis, you may find that Taoist philosophy can supplement your current beliefs. Why? Although devout followers of some religions may disagree, many will also point out that most belief systems are just different paths to the top of the mountain. At the summit, the view is the same no matter how you get there.

Understanding the basic principles of Taoism can enhance your T'ai Chi practice, particularly a solid understanding of the concept of yin and yang (see Chapter 3).

One favorite and lighthearted reading is *The Tao of Pooh*, by Benjamin Hoff, and another simple reading is *Tao Te Ching*, translated by Stephen Mitchell. Look for information in the Appendix to help you find them. Both are remarkably accessible introductions to Taoist thought, and you may want to read them regularly to remind yourself of Taoist principles and thoughts.

Watch T'ai Chi Videos

No, no, not kick-punch-ouch martial art movies, but instructional videos. Even after reading this book, taking a class, or watching one video, you can always pick up more by watching other teachers.

If you choose to study with a teacher, videos can help you with lessons in class. If you study on your own, videos can help expand your world with extra instruction. Every teacher has his or her own way of doing things. Be open-minded to these variations. Expose yourself to them gladly. Only with a broader view can you determine what is best for you.

One more thing: In addition to getting good stuff from videos, you can also find out what to avoid. There is no Worldwide Filtering Agency that allows only good practitioners or teachers to put themselves on the small screen. Nothing is sacred just because it's on video. So if something looks or feels really bad, it may be incorrect. Sometimes, observing glaring mistakes on a video can remind you to look for the same errors in your practice.

Peruse T'ai Chi Books

Okay, so now you're convinced to watch some T'ai Chi videos. Next comes printed matter. Books can be a valuable supplement to your practice, although finding out all you need to from one book (even this one!) is difficult. However, this book and others can be great resources and references as you progress along the path. From each book, you get explanations and insights from a different perspective that may broaden your understanding of T'ai Chi.

After you start establishing your own T'ai Chi library, you may find yourself thumbing through books just to pick out bits and pieces of wisdom. Guaranteed, every time you read one, you'll probably see something that you didn't see the time before! (See the Appendix for sources.)

Watch Yourself on Video

Just as watching sports on TV can be an enlightening way to pick up technique — good and bad! — watching yourself can be an eye-opener, too. "I really look like that?" Yep, the camera never lies. Especially if you are a visual person (and I truly am), seeing yourself do something that someone may have told you were doing can help you recognize it and realize that you need to change it. You just need to be a little merciless with yourself sometimes.

Try Meditating

Meditation, in some small way, is a part of every good T'ai Chi class or practice session. You can find some meditation exercises in Chapter 8 and also some Qigong meditations in Chapter 14. They aren't complicated. You don't need special candles or incense, and they are often done standing.

So what about the sitting meditations? They are another facet of a practice and are something you can try apart from your T'ai Chi session. You can find out more about the subject in *Meditation For Dummies* (published by Hungry Minds, Inc.).

Really, meditation isn't anything fancy, but is rather just a way to bring your mind to rest on a single thing for a period of time. One popular analogy is that meditation is like allowing a jar of muddy water to sit undisturbed on a shelf until the sediment settles and the water is clear. It gives you an opportunity to allow the chatter and clatter of daily life to subside, leaving you calmer and more relaxed. And best of all, it brings your attention into the present moment, allowing you to actually experience your life as it happens rather than daydreaming your life away.

Try this: On a chair or on the floor, sit in whatever way is comfortable so your body can relax. You can leave your eyes open or close them, whatever feels best to you. Simply take a few minutes to clear your mind. If a thought dances through your head (What's for dinner? What are the kids up to? What time is it?), acknowledge it and let it pass. You may find it helpful to focus on something, such as repeating a word, a phrase, a sound, your breathing, or even the flickering of a candle's light.

Practice Mentally

Great athletes visualize or mentally rehearse a game or technique as a part of training. You can do the same thing. Start by relaxing your mind with a little meditation. Then visualize yourself moving through a T'ai Chi movement or form.

You can use this technique to practice when you can't actually scoot around a room. For example, try it while standing in a long line, sitting in a waiting room, or during a boring office meeting (don't tell your boss I said that!).

Just close your eyes, relax your mind, and get moving mentally.

Dabble in Other Martial Arts

Even if you aren't studying T'ai Chi for self-defense purposes (and likely, you're not), if you understand the intent behind each movement, you'll be better able to think yourself through proper alignment and therefore get the most benefit. Reading books, studying with teachers of other martial arts styles, or even watching a few Jackie Chan movies (really!) can enhance your practice and open your mind to additional applications of your T'ai Chi techniques. Manny started in Tae Kwon Do and studied Hsing-I Chuan prior to his T'ai Chi studies. Any dedicated practice can develop discipline and inner peace.

One word, though: If you decide to pursue some combative martial arts, you should probably select one style as your major style. Other styles can add flavor but should not take practice time away from your major form, for example, T'ai Chi. Perfecting one style is difficult enough (and no one but the greatest masters can ever really claim to do that!).

Remember: The hunter who chases two rabbits will catch neither.

Push Against the Wall

Manny swears by this technique, although his colleagues may look the other way when they see him pushing against a wall while alone in a room. But, seriously, you can check out your stances and postures using the wall as a guide to help you identify and correct deficiencies in your body alignment.

Pick one "pushing" stance within a form. For example, try Single Whip (see Chapter 10). Put your right hand in a Dropped Hand position to your side and put your left hand out to your side, palm out as if pushing against an imaginary foe. But instead of pushing against a foe, place your left palm on a wall, tree, telephone pole, or some other solid object. In the position, push gently. Then focus on your feet and move your focus up through your body muscle-by-muscle and joint-by-joint. Inventory your body for muscle tension or for places where you begin to sort of clamp down or bind up. Relax these areas when you find them; then continue upward to your head and out through your arms. Don't forget your face!

It was said of the ancient T'ai Chi masters that their punches moved only a little and were not flashy or flamboyant, but they felt like mountains falling down on their opponents.

Stand on Bricks

Say what? Yes, I can see why this exercise may sound a little like a gardener trying to reach the top of the hedge. But this is *T'ai Chi For Dummies,* not *Gardening For Dummies,* so be reassured that I mean what I say.

Standing on the long side of bricks (one under each foot) quickly shows you if your balance is off or uneven, because the bricks can be a little unstable. Do this drill if you don't have bad knees, ankles, a low-back problem, or other problems that can be made worse if you fall off the bricks. And do it on a soft surface, too.

This drill is recommended by T'ai Chi Master Dr. Yang Jwing-Ming:

1. **While in the T'ai Chi Stance (see Chapter 8 for a reminder on proper alignment), place two bricks on their long narrow sides under your feet. The wider faces of the bricks should face each other and be parallel.**

2. **Let your weight sink straight down through your feet into the ground.**

If you are standing and sinking properly, the bricks stay put. You know pretty quickly if you aren't balanced, because the bricks roll inward or outward, forcing you to take a step off of one or the other or both. Pay attention to which leg (and to which direction) you roll off, because that's where you need balance and stance practice. For example, if a brick rolls inward, the leg is pressing inward. If it rolls outward, the leg is pressing outward.

Now, go stand on some bricks!

Pick up the Pace

T'ai Chi is mostly taught and practiced at a very slow tempo. But after all, T'ai Chi *is* a martial art at its core. So after you know the forms well and are able to perform them very, very slowly, try doing them a little faster and see if you can keep good balance, flow, and alignment.

Make sure that you really know the form well before you try to speed up. And I do mean well. Manny spent three years (yes, *three!*) practicing slowly before he could do them correctly at a faster pace.

Take this increase in steps. Don't go from molasses-in-January speed to race-horse tempo. Just pick it up a little a first. When that goes well and feels comfortable, pick it up a little more. You may spend days or weeks at one speed before moving on, though.

Moving faster will likely make you tense up your muscles again. So practice keeping them loose. You need to be able to work through a form at a speed without clamping down on your muscles before you move on.

Sheesh, how many warnings do we need? Here's another one: Moving faster means slightly more risk of twisting something — particularly if you tense up. So be sure to warm up thoroughly before trying a faster routine.

Apply T'ai Chi Principles to Everything You Do

There are opportunities to put a little T'ai Chi practice into practically everything you do. See Chapter 16 for more about that. Here are a few physical ways:

- ✔ Sink a little and do some abdominal breathing when stuck in a line at the bank or grocery store.

- ✔ Write T'ai Chi-style. Grasp the pen or pencil with the least amount of amount of force necessary.

- ✔ Drive with a relaxed grip on the steering wheel rather than white-knuckling your way down the road.

- ✔ Pull doors open by shifting your weight rather than pulling with your arms.

See what I mean? Then you've got the mental and mindful side:

✔ Pause mindfully at a red light and enter the present moment. It becomes an opportunity rather than just another dang obstacle to getting to your destination in a hurry.

✔ Try a mini-meditation while on hold on the phone.

Practice yielding and see how relaxed you feel and how much more efficient in life you actually become.

Chapter 23

Ten Things to Tell Yourself about Your Practice

In This Chapter

▶ Nagging yourself to a better practice and mindset

▶ Finding out some things to say to yourself

▶ Discovering that the journey itself is the goal

*W*hether you're preparing for a job interview, trying to memorize a speech, or going through couples therapy, you should always keep telling yourself little things to keep yourself on track.

This is where I list those little nagging phrases and reminders. If you've read part of the book already, you may recognize them. If not, consider this list a preview. As you take on a T'ai Chi practice to whatever extent, you should tell yourself all of these things over and over. Maybe that means writing the ones you need most on a scrap of paper and sticking them to your bathroom mirror or car dashboard. Maybe that means doodling them on a notepad during a boring meeting or class. Maybe that means just pestering yourself as you start and practice your forms.

Just keep telling yourself the following things. Nag, nag, nag . . .

Slow Down

I feel like a broken record. Oops, dating myself. Let's see, like a CD with a scratch? Translation: You hear it again and again. And if you tell yourself nothing else, tell this to yourself again and again: Slow down. Slow down more. Slow down even more.

This is indeed a cardinal principal of T'ai Chi practice. Slow down physically; slow down mentally. Let the relaxed movements of your body calm your mind, and let the peaceful thought patterns influence your body's movements.

Life gallops along at an incredibly fast pace compared to the pace of just a few years ago. Be honest — you probably get frustrated when the driver in front of you moves at a more, uh, *relaxed* pace than you want. But maybe the driver in front of you has figured out that putting on the brakes can help life become more fruitful and healthy.

As the Buddhist saying goes, "Life is so short that it must be lived very slowly."

This Is Not a Competition

It really isn't, you know. No matter how much and how hard you practice, there is always be someone better, there is always one more move to perfect (as if perfection is possible? See the next thing to tell yourself!), or there is always another form you can take lower or push farther. So stop competing, stop comparing yourself to the next, stop watching yourself in the mirror, and just get on with practicing the forms.

By the same token, there is always someone worse. But what does that mean, really? You're just farther along in your practice, which doesn't really matter. The only comparison that matters is the one with yourself.

The best teachers are the most humble and modest ones, very often the ones you may casually meet who never tell you how they are the best — because, well, it doesn't matter. They just practice. Whenever Manny, my collaborator and T'ai Chi teacher, receives a compliment on his abilities, he finds himself mumbling about how his teacher is so much better than him. Of course, his teacher would also humbly point out that he knows nothing compared to *his* teacher. And so the progression goes.

It's not about being better than others; it's about becoming a better you.

I Can Never Be Perfect

The word "perfect" and the art of T'ai Chi don't belong in the same room, let alone the same sentence. In T'ai Chi, you can always learn more, improve physically or mindfully, or incorporate the principles of practice more thoroughly into your daily life.

Perfection, as the world thinks of it, just isn't possible. Does a gourmet chef ever stop tinkering with his or her signature dish? Does a painter ever look at a piece of artwork and not want to just change one little stroke? Does a writer ever read something he or she thinks is the best it can be, and not find something to change? (I answer that last one with a resounding "no.")

So, forget trying to be perfect and just be.

My Journey Is the Goal

The harder and more single-mindedly you focus on your goal, the longer it can take you to achieve because you forget about the necessary learning process along the way.

Life is what happens while we are waiting for something to happen. Don't worry about what you can accomplish in T'ai Chi, when you can accomplish it, or whether you should do something differently to accomplish it. Just enjoy the journey, and the benefits come naturally.

As Coach John Madden told his Oakland Raiders before an important game, "Don't worry about the horse being blind, just load the wagon." I don't really know what that means, but it sounds like a cool phrase that fits here.

It's a Cumulative Thing

You've heard of so-called overnight sensations in music or movies — artists who actually spend a lifetime paying their dues before they become an overnight sensation. The same goes for T'ai Chi, where accomplishment comes after repeated steady effort over a long period of time of correct practice steeped in all the principles.

You must practice simply to practice — correctly of course — not with one eye fixed upon a certain goal, because the accumulation of your good practice is what leads to being more accomplished.

In Manny's case, he practiced T'ai Chi diligently for several hours almost daily for a year and a half, never really "feeling" it but sticking with it. Then, one day, during a performance of the Yang Long Form, his hands suddenly "came to life" and felt very "full" — full of energy. He was finally moving chi into his hands, but it took months and months of accumulated practice, with full attention to the principles.

Snow that slides off a heavily laden branch is the result of an accumulation of snow, which has gathered one tiny flake at a time until the load reaches the point of sliding off. Likewise, with your T'ai Chi practice, every practice session is another snowflake, and over time, the accumulated and sound practice sessions will deliver the benefits you seek.

T'ai Chi Is a Martial Art

No matter what your reasons for studying and practicing T'ai Chi, remember that its essence is still a system born for self-defense. The difference between T'ai Chi's martial principles and other fighting and attacking forms — is that it places a premium on yielding, flowing, and avoidance of conflict. No high-flying leaps or smashing through bricks and boards with the fists. Nevertheless, T'ai Chi is a remarkably effective system of self-defense because it does not place a premium on muscular strength. Legends abound of older T'ai Chi practitioners defeating younger attackers, or even of one master defeating several opponents at once — because the victor knew how to flow with the right energy and not rely on brute strength.

Even if you practice for health reasons, keep the martial intent of each movement in mind as you perform them to help you align your body properly. For example, remembering that a hand or foot is placed so you are better blocked from an opponent helps you remember the form better than if you just memorize steps. Plus, the strategic placements are designed to optimize energy (chi) flow.

Enjoy Any Losses

Now, if this line were coming from your banker or stockbroker, you'd be looking for a new one ASAP. But it's coming from a T'ai Chi book. T'ai Chi is a martial art, but not an aggressive one. T'ai Chi derives its strength from the ability to yield in the face of an attack. If an aggressor pushes you and expects resistance but finds none, the aggressor's balance gets thrown off, which means that you can more easily deal with the big meanie. So let yourself "lose" in some situations to give yourself a really big win in others. You can read more about the principle and concepts of pushing and yielding in Chapter 6.

Letting yourself lose applies to your personal interactions in daily life as well. The winner of an argument between a husband and wife isn't always the real winner. Sometimes, just letting go and "losing" can make you a true winner, both in your relationship and with your health.

No, no, I'm not telling you to roll over and play dead in life. Yes, yes, some things are worth standing up for. But you have to pick your battles carefully. Whether you have to wait an extra five minutes in a restaurant or you complain that the toothpaste tube is squeezed in the middle or from the end, winning isn't worth the bother of a battle.

There Are Lessons to Learn In Everything I Do

Every experience in your life and every person you encounter carry the potential to teach you something. Manny recalls this really wonderful quote (which he thought came from Ralph Waldo Emerson, though he's not sure, but what does it matter, really?): "I reckon every man is my master in that I can learn something from him."

Dealing with so-called difficult people are opportunities to negotiate in new ways, to think about how you can deal with different situations, and to overcome and stay calm in petty encounters. Maybe it's your mother or mother-in-law with whom you always seem to get into tiffs. Think about what they're saying and the feelings they are expressing as a way to discover more about what you are feeling in response and, in turn, how you can change these feelings — or even how you are affecting the other person's feelings.

Everyone can find out more about his or her true nature in the face of conflict or inconvenience than when everything is going hunky-dory.

I Am a Teacher, Too

If you are sincere in your T'ai Chi practice, your life will change.

Whoa, that's heavy stuff. But it's true. A true practitioner develops calm, patience, and the ability to see the world with a broader vision, as well as the ability to respond to potential conflicts without first exploding. These qualities will slowly become apparent to the people in your life. And with that, you become a teacher. Others — if perceptive and indeed ready to learn — can find out how to do the same in their own lives.

But these changes are all very subtle. You don't prance around telling everybody to watch you, to see how great you are, and to do what you do. Just do. Just be. And the teaching and learning will happen.

As James Allen wrote in *As a Man Thinketh,* calm is like a shade-giving tree that people seek out.

My Path Is Not the Only One

T'ai Chi — especially your style or practice of T'ai Chi — is not the only way to the top of the mountain. T'ai Chi is not better than Yoga, or meditation, or Qigong. For some, it is better. For others, it may not be.

Ranking exercise programs or belief systems isn't necessary, because everybody is different and what is an A+ to one person may be a D- to another. Different things appeal to different people and effect people differently. If it works for you, it just works. And that's great.

In *The Teachings of Don Juan*, author Carlos Castaneda writes that there are many paths to follow, and everyone should try out as many paths as they can to find the path that "has heart." That's what this journey is about — experimenting to find your path with heart — whether you choose T'ai Chi or another movement form. If you're listening and feeling, you'll recognize the path when you find it.

As the saying goes, "There are many paths to the top of the mountain, but when you get there, the view is the same."

Chapter 24

Ten Wise Taoist Lessons

T'ai Chi is heavily steeped in Taoist philosophy. So knowing the basics about how to live that philosophy can give your T'ai Chi practice a real boost. And knowing the why and wherefore behind a form can help you do it better!

Even if you decide that you aren't interested in undertaking a deep study of Taoism and you aren't interested in the religious facets of Taoism, take a look through these 10 tempting lessons. They can not only give you some insights into the thinking of Taoism and the practice of T'ai Chi, but they can also help you live a calmer and fuller life, whatever your own beliefs may be.

Weigh Your Wu Wei

The phrase "wu wei" (*woo* way) translates loosely into something like "effort-less effort" or "do without doing." Wait a minute, to do something you have to *do* something? So what is this "without doing" stuff? Westerners tend to *do* harder than they need to most of the time — force the lid off the jar, jam the car into the smallest parking space, pound harder on the keyboard, lift too much weight in the gym, and so on. Really, wu wei's lesson is to stop doing so hard, to go with the flow, to let it happen — basically, to stop forcing life to be the way you want it to be right *now*.

If you ever get a chance to watch a T'ai Chi master in action, you'll notice that the master doesn't seem to be trying very hard, yet he is effectively moving an opponent. In some ways, the same thing can apply to other physical activities, such as the prima ballerina effortlessly gliding across the stage or a runner in the front of the pack floating along the course while the back-of-the-packer is straining, grunting, and wheezing.

Take what the opponent (life) has given you to work with, and use it to your advantage.

Find Humility

The classic piece of Taoist literature, *Tao Te Ching*, advises readers to "be like water." What is it about water? Water always seeks to fill the lowest place. The ocean is lower than the rivers, so the waters of the rivers flow into it. And yet the ocean, even in its lowest position, is the strongest. So if you're like water, you'll be powerfully humble, seeking lower positions, yet commanding others who still seek higher positions.

Humility serves two purposes:

✔ To remind you that someone will always be better than you, be it in T'ai Chi practice, your bowling league, a gin rummy club, or your company's department.

✔ To keep you from going around blabbing and boasting about how good you are. Ever notice how the best of the best, the real masters, never tell you that? They let their actions speak for themselves. And if someone doesn't know that you're the best, he or she is less likely to try to knock you down a notch or two.

Be Soft and Supple

In Stephen Mitchell's translation of the classic Taoist literature, *Tao Te Ching*, he writes:

Men are born soft and supple; dead, they are stiff and hard. Thus whoever is stiff and inflexible is a disciple of death. Whoever is soft and yielding is a disciple of life. The hard and stiff will be broken. The soft and supple will prevail.

The lesson? Try to remain soft and supple, not only physically but also mentally — in word and in action. Would you try to tackle and topple the NFL's leading blocker who weights 350 pounds or so? I doubt it. You'd scramble, duck, cover, and maneuver; therefore, you'd yield to superior force.

Yearn for Yin and Yang

Everything in the world has a complementary opposite — for example, salt and pepper, oil and vinegar, Mutt and Jeff, and Dr. Jekyll and Mr. Hyde. These duos aren't made up for no reason; they're like yin and yang, and you can't have one without the other. I discuss yin and yang in more depth in Chapter 3.

Hence, another saying: "Pleasure and pain are like two bells hanging beside each other in a temple garden. You cannot ring one without causing the other to vibrate a little." The yin-yang symbol reminds you that life is made up of opposites and that life is a continuous cycle of these opposites. Good times follow bad, sun follows rain, and smiles follow tears. So when times are good, you cherish them, partly because of their impermanence. And when times are bad, you don't worry too much, because you know that they can't last forever.

Sense "The Uncarved Block"

The Chinese word "p'u" (sounds like *put* without the *t* at the end) translates loosely into "the uncarved block" or, less abstractly put, "things in their natural state." This is meant to remind you against trying too hard to figure things out or trying to use brute force to make things happen.

How many times does your rational mind get in the way of your true visceral understanding? It's much easier to stop trying to make things into something they aren't and accept their "natural state."

As a teen-ager, when something didn't go as I wanted it to go, my mom or dad would invariably say something annoyingly parental: "Guess it wasn't meant to be." Boy, did that tick me off! I mean, if I wanted it to be, dang it, it should be, right? As I grew older (and, sigh, yes, wiser . . . thanks Mom and Dad), I stopped trying so hard, learning unwittingly about "the uncarved block."

Benjamin Hoff, in *The Tao of Pooh,* writes, "Pooh can't explain the Uncarved Block. He just *is* it." (Find information about this fine book in the Appendix.)

Let Emptiness Be

The Western mind sees emptiness as something negative, an absence of something. However, enjoy for a moment how the Eastern mind sees emptiness — as something very positive. Why? Because Eastern philosophy says that the empty space is what makes a cup useful (what good is a cup that is filled in?) or that the empty space of a doorway is what allows you to enter a room.

Meditation is a practice aimed at "emptying the mind." It unclutters the mind and leaves some space to bring in new thoughts.

The common analogy that my collaborator Manny likes to cite: "Your mind is like a jar of clear water. All day long, things happen to cloud your mind, like putting dirt into the jar of water and stirring it around. Meditation, then, is like putting the jar onto a shelf and letting it sit undisturbed, allowing the sediment to settle so the water again becomes clear."

Another story about Zen tradition for the road:

A European philosophy professor goes to visit a Zen master. After listening to the professor ramble on at length about how much the professor already knows about Zen, the Zen master begins to pour his visitor a cup of tea, not stopping when the liquid reaches the brim. The tea starts to flow over the side of the cup, but the master keeps pouring.

"Master, the cup is full; no more can go in!" the professor finally says.

"So is your mind," the Master replies. "How can I put anything in unless you are willing to empty your cup?"

Seek Simplicity

When all is said and done, life is simple. You live, you learn, you seek happiness and love, you get old, and you die.

Whether in T'ai Chi practice, at work, in personal relationships, or shopping at the mall, live and act simply and truthfully. Get out of your own way, and you'll be amazed how many of your problems resolve themselves.

Center Yourself

Too much of even a good thing can be bad. The lesson at its core? Live moderately and avoid extremes.

In T'ai Chi movement, you find out how to avoid reaching out to an extreme, straightening an elbow or a knee to an extreme, and pushing your weight to one side to an extreme — all of which can upset your balance. Where does the high wire walker hold onto the pole? In the center, of course. That's where the best balance is found.

Not only as a T'ai Chi practitioner do you avoid extremes of movement, but as a human being, you are best to avoid extremes of emotion. Does this mean becoming apathetic and floating through life? Not at all! Does this mean not feeling? Oh my, no! It means looking at things calmly rather than just flying off the handle.

Practice Personal Patience

The value of patience can't be valued enough, both in T'ai Chi practice and in life.

I return to those aggravating parental sayings. You've heard them, I know. As a teen-ager, when you were cautioned to "be patient" about getting something, you wanted to explode. You wanted it "now!"

Patience is about taking the time needed to get a T'ai Chi movement right and, at the same time, knowing that getting it right is not a matter of life or death. Manny, my trusty collaborator and T'ai Chi instructor, recalls a student who once said to him: "I'll get this move right if it takes all day and all night!" With that lack of patience, it didn't take long for the student to wear out and give up. He soon quit the class in frustration.

Really, impatience is a carryover of what infects you in everyday life. Ask yourself: "How many times do I get impatient and perhaps curse a little when I get behind someone walking or driving slower than I want to go?"

In T'ai Chi, then, patience is king: Having a form down pat after a few repetitions isn't possible. Manny says that any number of people ask him on the first day of class, "How long is it going to take to learn T'ai Chi?" His rather smarty pants (but true!) answer is "As soon as I learn it, I'll let you know."

Live in the Present Moment

This lesson comes quite naturally after the lesson of patience. That's because of a lot of our hurry-hurry comes from wanting to be someplace, anyplace, other than where we are — or simply wanting life in general to move more quickly.

As a young man, Manny says that he worked a summer job in the rice fields of south Louisiana. One day, he said, "Ah! Come on, make it quitting time!" The foreman looked at him and said, "Son, don't ever wish for your life to pass faster than it already does."

I remember nearly being in tears upon college graduation. Why? Because I had a rather prestigious fellowship to study in Europe for a year. But that wasn't why I was upset. I was upset thinking that because I waited another year to go and then would spend a year abroad, I would be so far behind all my fellow journalism graduates, many of whom were already moving on into nice jobs at daily newspapers. One of my favorite professors, coddling a whiskey in that curmudgeon journalist way, looked at me and said, "You will have 40 years to work. Go! Go have fun, and go learn!" Begrudgingly, I did. And I am truly thankful for taking that moment as it came to me.

Henry David Thoreau once said, "Only that day dawns to which we are fully awake."

Chapter 25

Ten Quotes to Live By

In This Chapter

▶ Collecting cool quotes

▶ Flowing and fathoming philosophy

▶ Integrating wisdom into your life

*O*ne beautiful and thought-provoking part of studying T'ai Chi is discovering all the quotes and pieces of wisdom. You can probably take any example in this list and think on it for days, if not years. You can analyze it, take it apart, put it together, and still not have it fully figured out. You'll still have enough to mull over for another lifetime.

Some of these quotes aren't taken directly from classical T'ai Chi literature, but they are just as applicable to practicing T'ai Chi principles, which are essentially the principles of life.

So without any explanation to contaminate your own thought process, here are ten wise quotes from which to live and learn.

Discover Yourself

Wanting to reform the world without discovering one's true self is like trying to cover the world with leather to avoid the pain of walking on stones and thorns. It is much simpler to wear shoes.

—Ramana Maharshi

Be Soft and Yielding

Men are born soft and supple; dead, they are stiff and hard. Plants are born tender and pliant; dead, they are brittle and dry. Thus, whoever is stiff and inflexible is a disciple of death. Whoever is soft and yielding is a disciple of life. The hard and stiff will be broken. The soft and supple will prevail.

—Lao Tzu, *Tao Te Ching*, translated by Stephen Mitchell

Live Slowly

Life is so short that it must be lived very slowly.

—Buddhist saying

Have a Mind Like a Mirror

The mind of a perfect man is like a mirror. It grasps nothing. It expects nothing. It reflects but does not hold. Therefore, the perfect man can act without effort.

—Chuang-Tzu, *The Writings of Chuang-Tzu*

Be Still

Self-control is strength; right thought is mastery; calmness is power; say unto your heart, "Peace, be still."

—James Allen, *As a Man Thinketh*

Gently Overcome the Rigid

Nothing in the world is as soft and yielding as water. Yet for dissolving the hard and inflexible, nothing can surpass it. The soft overcomes the hard; the gentle overcomes the rigid. Everyone knows this is true, but few can put it into practice. Therefore the Master remains serene in the midst of sorrow.

—Lao Tzu, *Tao Te Ching*, translated by Stephen Mitchell

Flow Ultimately

Flow with whatever may happen and let your mind be free: Stay centered by accepting what you are doing. This is the ultimate.

—Chuang-Tzu, *The Writings of Chuang-Tzu*

Look Inside If You Miss The Mark

The inferior archer, when he misses the mark, first looks for blame in his bow. The superior archer first looks for blame in himself.

—Traditional saying of *Kyudo* (Japanese archery)

Stay Strong and Gentle

It is the weak who are cruel: gentleness can only be expected from the strong.

—Leo Rosten, quoted by Leo Buscaglia

Begin Your Journey with One Step

The journey of a thousand miles begins with but a single step.

—Various Buddhist and Taoist sources

Appendix

• w w w . e a s t w e s t q i . c o m • • • • • • •

*I*n this appendix, I list a variety of resources you may want to explore under four different headings:

✔ **Finding instruction and networking:** This section is where you can find resources for classes, instructors, videos/audiotapes, and other instruction, as well as contacts for organizations and associations through which you may find teachers or other information about instruction. Don't miss each group's Web site, most of which often have links to many other resources; these sites aren't listed separately under "Surfing the Web."

✔ **Hitting the library:** If you want to do more reading, here's where you find information about selected books, journals, and magazines.

✔ **Surfing the Web:** This is a section listing Web sites that aren't associated with a group or other resource listed separately in this appendix. Many are full of education and links. *Note:* Web sites sometimes change names or come and go. If an address I list doesn't exist, do a search in your favorite search engine for the organization's name to see whether the page has moved.

✔ **Getting equipped:** Look for contacts here to catalogs, equipment, clothing, and other accessories you may want for your exercise and practice.

T'ai Chi Chuan and Qigong

Finding instruction and networking

Bingkun Hu, master Qigong instructor. Holds regular weekend classes. Instructional videotape, *12 Qigong Treasures for Beginners* (1999). 2114 Sacramento St., Berkeley, CA 94702; phone: 510-841-6810.

East West Academy of Healing Arts, a Qigong association that offers seminars, conference, news, and other education. www.eastwestqi.com

Manny Fuentes, a master instructor and clinical exercise physiologist offering classes, lectures, and workshops for health professionals and the public. P.O. Box 53464, Lafayette, LA 70505; phone: 337-289-7358. Mannyfuentes@hotmail.com

The Qigong Institute, a non-profit educational and research institute and resource for teachers. Good place to find other information and links or referrals. Kenneth Sancier, founder. 561 Berkeley Ave., Menlo Park, CA 94025; phone: 415-323-1221. www.qigonginstitute.org

Hitting the library

Applied Tai Chi Chuan by Nigel Sutton. Boston, MA: Charles E. Tuttle Co., Inc., 1991.

Beginning T'ai Chi by Tri Thong Dang. Rutland, VT, and Tokyo, Japan: Charles E. Tuttle Company, 1994.

Chi Kung: Health and Martial Arts by Dr. Yang Jwing-Ming. Jamaica Plain, MA: YMAA Publication Center, 1985.

The Complete Book of Tai Chi Chuan: A comprehensive guide to principles and practice by Wong Kiew Kit. Rockport, MA: Element Books, 1996. Also includes a section on Qigong.

The Dao of Taijiquan: Way to Rejuvenation by Jou, Tsung Hwa. Riscataway, NJ: Tai Chi Foundation, 1998.

How to Grasp the Bird's Tail If You Don't Speak Chinese by Jane Schorre. Berkeley, CA: North Atlantic Books, 2000. An entertaining little book that helps dissect what all the calligraphy and characters mean and why they are translated as they are.

Qigong for Beginners: Eight Easy Movements For Vibrant Health by Stanley D. Wilson. Portland, OR: Rudra Press, 1997.

Tai Chi Chuan: The philosophy of yin and yang and its application by Douglas Lee. Burbank, CA: O'Hara Publications, Inc., 1976.

Tai Chi Chuan & Qigong: Techniques & Training by Wolfgang Metzger and Peifang Zhou with Manfred Grosser. New York, NY: Sterling Publishing, 1996.

Tai Chi Chuan's Internal Secrets by Doc Fai-Wong and Jane Hallander. Burbank, CA: Unique Publications, 1991.

Tai Chi Classics by Waysun Liao. Boston, Mass: Shambhala Publications, Inc., 1990.

T'ai Chi for Two: The Practice of Push Hands by Paul Crompton. Boston, MA: Shambhala, 1989.

The Way of Qigong: The Art and Science of Chinese Energy Healing by Kenneth S. Cohen. New York, NY: Ballantine Books, 1997.

Yang Style Tai Chi Chuan by Dr. Yang Jwing-Ming. Hollywood, CA: Unique Publications, 1982.

Surfing the Web

New Age Directory, an online resource for finding associations, instruction, and links to other groups. www.newagedirectory.com/qigong.htm or www.newagedirectory.com/tai_chi.htm

Wayfarer Publications, an online catalog of T'ai Chi and Qigong books and videos. Also a guide to selecting videos for your needs, and subscription information for *Tai Chi Magazine*. www.tai-chi.com/catalog

Lee Scheele's Online Tai Chi Chuan. A collection of introductory writings, translations of the classics, definitions, and thoughts on T'ai Chi and on Chi itself. Plus an incredibly extensive links page. www.scheele.org/lee/taichi.html

General Mind-Body and Fitness Sources

Getting Connected

National Center for Complementary and Alternative Medicine, a division of the government's National Institutes of Health. Conducts and supports research and provides information to the public. A Web site now provides information about alternative health options. Click CAM on PubMed and search for a topic. Phone 888-644-6226. www.nccam.nih.gov

Hitting the library

365 Tao: Daily Meditations by Deng Ming-Dao. San Francisco, CA: HarperSanFrancisco, 1992.

The Healer Within: The Four Essential Self-Care Techniques for Optimal Health by Roger O.M.D. Jahnke. San Francisco, CA: Harper, 1997.

Meditation For Dummies by Stephan Bodian. New York, NY: Hungry Minds, Inc., 1999.

Mind-Body Fitness For Dummies by Therese Iknoian. New York, NY: Hungry Minds, Inc., 2000.

Nutrition For Dummies by Carol Ann Rinzler. New York, NY: Hungry Minds, Inc., 1999.

The Relaxation Response by Herbert Benson. Boston, MA: G.K. Hall, 1975.

Somatics: Reawakening the Mind's Control of Movement, Flexibility, and Health by Thomas Hanna. Reading, MA: Addison-Wesley, 1988.

Tao of Pooh by Benjamin Hoff. New York, NY: E.P. Dutton, 1982

Tao Te Ching: A New English Version by Stephen Mitchell. New York, NY: HarperPerennial, 1991.

Zen in the Martial Arts by Joe Hyams. New York: St. Martin's Press, 1979.

Surfing the Web

American Dietetic Association: Another useful Web site for helping out with healthy eating. www.eatright.org

American Heart Association: Gives you tips on nutrition and exercise. www.americanheart.org

Mind-Body Medical Institute. Harvard Physician Herbert Benson — the person who coined the term "relaxation response" — has a site full of news, research, and education. www.mindbody.harvard.edu

Total Fitness Network: Web site of general fitness and training advice from Therese Iknoian, author of *Mind-Body Fitness For Dummies* and *T'ai Chi For Dummies.* www.totalfitnessnetwork.com

Getting Equipped

Living Arts, Yoga and mind-body props, clothing, accessories, and instructional video tapes, including tapes by Patricia Walden, John Friend, and Rodney Lee. Phone 877-989-6321. www.livingarts.com or www.gaiam.com

Planet Earth Music, producer and distributor of music appropriate for mind-body arts. Phone 800-825-8656. www.planet-earth-music.com

Index

● ●

• **F** •

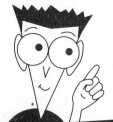

FOR DUMMIES®

The easy way to get more done and have more fun

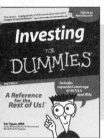
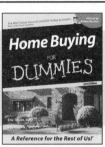
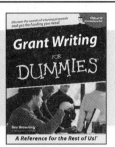
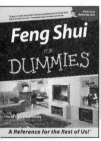
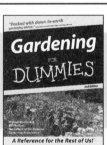
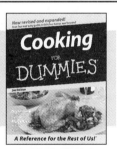
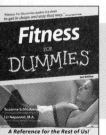
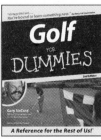
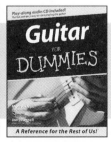
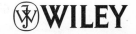

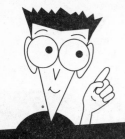
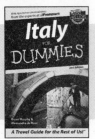
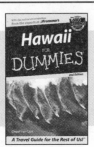
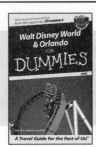
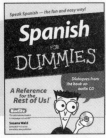
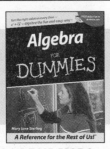
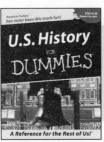
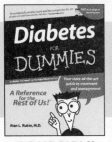
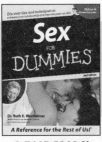
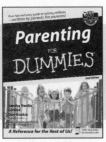

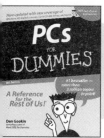
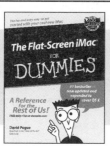
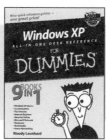
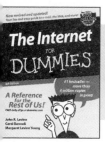
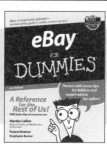
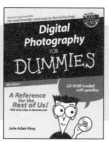
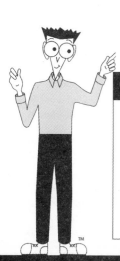

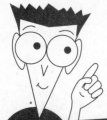
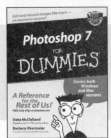
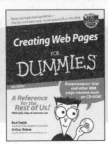
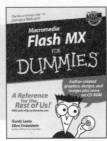
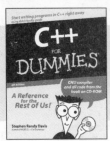
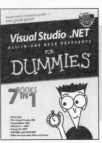
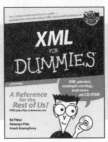
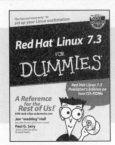
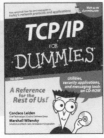
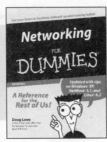
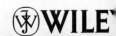